THE DIABETES IMPROVEMENT PROGRAM

the ultimate handbook for using foods & supplements
to slow and reverse the complications of diabetes

by Patrick Quillin, PhD,RD,CNS

The Leader Co., Inc.
North Canton, Ohio

Other books by Patrick Quillin (website: www.4nutrition.com)
-BEATING CANCER WITH NUTRITION, Nutrition Times Press, Tulsa,1998
-THE HEALING POWER OF CAYENNE PEPPER, Leader Co.,Inc., Canton, 1998
-KITCHEN HEALTH TIPS (video), Nutrition Times Press, Tulsa, 1997
-HEALING SECRETS FROM THE BIBLE, Nutrition Times Press, Tulsa, 1996
-HONEY, GARLIC & VINEGAR, Leader Co., Inc., N. Canton, OH, 1996
-HEALING POWER OF WHOLE FOODS, Vitamix, Cleveland, 1994
-ADJUVANT NUTRITION IN CANCER TREATMENT, Cancer Treatment Research Foundation, Arlington Heights, IL, 1994
-AMISH FOLK MEDICINE, Leader Co.,Inc., N.Canton, OH, 1993
-SAFE EATING, M.Evans, NY, 1990
-THE LA COSTA BOOK OF NUTRITION, Pharos Books, New York, 1988
-HEALING NUTRIENTS, Contemporary Books, Chicago, 1987
-THE LA COSTA PRESCRIPTION FOR LONGER LIFE, Ballantine, NY, 1985

DIABETES IMPROVEMENT PROGRAM available exclusively from:
The Leader Co., Inc., 931 N. Main #101, N.Canton, OH 44720
ph.330-494-6988, fax 494-6989;website:www.booksforhealth.com

TELL US YOUR STORY
We want to hear your experiences about using nutrition as part of your diabetes treatment. Please send us your personal experience with an address or phone number on how to contact you. Your story may provide hope and inspiration for others suffering from the same condition. Thank you.

Printed in Canada

CONTENTS

DEDICATION
My utmost admiration and appreciation go forth to the bold physicians and healers throughout history who were more concerned with their patient's welfare than peer approval.

ACKNOWLEDGEMENTS
Thanks to my wife, Noreen, for her stellar work in creating the wonderful chapter in this book of nutritious and delicious recipes for you, the reader, to feast on.

EXECUTIVE SUMMARY

"Natural forces within us are the true healers." Hippocrates, *father of modern medicine, circa 400 BC*

      If you are too tired to read this entire book, then please read this short summary to get you started. Once you are under a doctor's care for your diabetes, then please do the following basic steps to get your health moving in the right direction:

♥ DETERMINATION. Have a firm conviction that you can improve your health through lifestyle changes such as diet, exercise, and supplements. <u>You can make a difference</u> in the outcome of your diabetes.

♥ LOSE WEIGHT. Gradually begin a weight loss program. 90% of Type 2 diabetics are obese. Weight loss usually brings considerable improvements in blood glucose regulation and, for some people, return to a healthy weight brings complete remission of the diabetes.

♥ EAT WHOLESOME NATURAL FOODS. Eat a diet of natural unprocessed foods. Shop the perimeter of the grocery store where you will find fresh fruits and vegetables, chicken, turkey, fish, meat, eggs, and bread. Venture into the "deep dark interior" of your grocery store only to get sacks of dried beans and brown rice.

♥ RATIO OF MACRONUTRIENTS. Mix your food in ratio of about 25% protein, 25% fat, and 50% complex high fiber carbohydrates. This means that looking at your dinner plate, you need to have about 1/3 of the plate covered with lean and clean protein food, such as chicken, turkey, fish, lean beef, pork, or beans. Another 1/3 of your plate needs to be covered with cooked plant foods, such as beans, vegetables, bread, squash, potatoes. The remaining 1/3 of your plate needs to be uncooked and unprocessed plant foods, such as a tossed salad of fresh colorful vegetables. Include the superfoods of brewer's yeast, flax oil, cinnamon, garlic, vinegar, onions, and fish in your diet often.

♥ Drink at least 8 cups of clean water daily.

♥ Get 30 minutes of exercise daily. Brisk walking is the most realistic, since you can do it without a partner, anywhere, anytime.

♥ Take the following nutritional supplements on a daily basis: 500 mg vitamin C, 500 mg niacin (inositol hexanicatinate), 50 mg B-6, 600 mcg B-12, 400 iu vitamin E (mixed tocopherols), 300 mg magnesium citrate, 300 mg sulfur (methyl sulfonyl methane), 6 mg manganese, 10 mg zinc (picolinate), 2 mg vanadyl sulfate, 400 mcg chromium picolinate, 100 mg lipoic acid, 100 mg L-carnitine, essential fatty acids of 1000 mg EPA and 250 mg GLA, 200 mg gymnema sylvestre, 200 mg bitter melon extract, 100 mg ginseng. You can buy these items individually at your local health food store.

♥ If you will adhere to the program outlined in this book, then the Type 2 diabetic can expect to find the following benefits: better control of blood sugar, lower ketones and more energy, better wound healing, better eyesight and lowered risk for eye complications, better circulation to the feet and hands and reversal of "numbness" and neuropathies, lowered fats in the blood to prevent heart disease, lowered risk for kidney damage, improvement in mental and physical energy levels including memory and alertness.

CHAPTER 1

UNDERSTANDING DIABETES
A MODERN EPIDEMIC

"Sugar is without question the number one murderer in the history of humanity." Sakurazawa, Japanese author of 50 books on natural healing, 1964

HOW IS THIS BOOK GOING TO HELP YOU, THE DIABETIC READER?

No one with a headache is suffering from a deficiency of aspirin. And the vast majority of Type 2 diabetics do not have a deficiency of insulin. Their entire blood glucose regulatory mechanisms are malfunctioning. This book is going to give you the tools to understand how diabetes begins, what are the underlying causes, and how to make reasonable changes

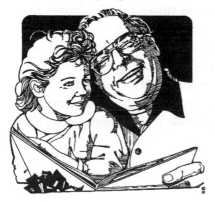

in your lifestyle that beat diabetes with nutrition. This DIABETES IMPROVEMENT PROGRAM can have a huge impact in your quality and quantity of life and prevention of the common complications of diabetes, such as eye, kidney, nerve, and heart problems. This book shares with you the secrets of a handful of "superfoods" to add to your daily diet, some examples of nutritious and delicious foods to control blood glucose, a few inexpensive nutrition supplements, the importance of 30 minutes a day of exercise, and the crucial therapy of reaching your ideal body weight.

With this clinically proven, scientifically validated, logical, and inexpensive program, you will find a new level of vigor that you haven't felt in years. If you follow the recommendations in this book, then it will likely add years to your life and life to your years.

DOES LIFESTYLE OR GENETICS CAUSE DIABETES?

The Pima Indians of the Southwestern United States can help us answer this question. A physician who worked with the Pima Indians found 1 case of diabetes among the entire Pima tribe in the year 1908, which was around the time that these Native Americans began to embrace the "western" diet of highly refined carbohydrates and sugar. When Dr. Elliott Joslin, founder of the Joslin Clinic, visited these Pima Indians in 1937, he identified 21 diabetics. In 1954, Drs. Parks and Waskow recorded 283 diabetics on the same reservation. By

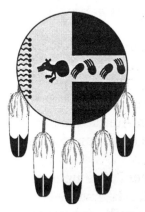

1965, there were 500 Pima diabetics. Today, nearly 60% of all Pima adults suffer from Type 2 diabetes. However, a splinter group of genetically similar Pima Indians living in New Mexico who did not embrace the western lifestyle of sugar, salt, fat, alcohol, obesity and sedentary lifestyle have an extremely low incidence of diabetes.[1] Most Pima Indians probably have a genetic vulnerability to diabetes that only surfaces when they eat the wrong foods and become obese through sedentary lifestyle. Most diseases, actually, are a collision between a genetic vulnerability and environmental insult.

Another example of the role played by lifestyle on diabetes involves the Yemenites from the Middle East who have lived in Israel for over 25 years and have a much higher incidence of diabetes than Yemenites who continued to consume the low sugar unrefined diet in their native land. The diet of both groups of Yemenites has similar calories, and ratios of protein, carbohydrates, and fats. The only difference in those Yemenites who have a much higher incidence of diabetes is the 20% of calories consumed from refined white sugar.[2]

Americans have also moved from various ancestral diets throughout the world that had almost no sugar to the "modern" diet of 20% of calories from sugar. We have suffered the consequences in deviating from our lifestyle that kept our ancestors alive. The incidence of diabetes has doubled over the past decade from 10 million to now 20 million Americans with diabetes, half of which don't even know that they have the disease. Diabetes is now one of the most rapidly growing diseases in America--primarily because of our poor diet and sedentary lifestyle.

Researchers now speculate that ancestral groups who have a "thrifty gene", or have been exposed to frequent periods of famines, are more vulnerable to diabetes. These people survived famines with the ability to conserve calories. Yet when food is abundantly available, as it is in America today, and these people get obese, this thrifty gene turns poor diet and obesity into diabetes.

The average American consumes over 700 doughnuts per year, much to the detriment of our health. Is it worth it? This book is about empowerment, not about guilt. It is about giving you back control of your life and health, not about finger pointing or blaming anyone.

CHANGING THE UNDERLYING CAUSES OF DIABETES.

What if I slammed my thumb in my desk drawer every morning for a week. The first time it happened, it really hurt. The next day I do it again and my thumb is swollen and painful. By the end of the week, my thumb is blue and red, bloody and swollen and very painful. So I go to Doctor A, who tells me he is going to inject my thumb with anti-inflammatory drugs to reduce the swelling. I get a second opinion from Doctor B who tells me that she wants to give me pain medication to better tolerate the discomfort. I get a third opinion from Doctor C who wants to cut off the thumb because it looks defective. The real cure here is to stop slamming my thumb in the desk drawer.

You may ask: "What does this example have to do with me beating my diabetes?" Let's look at the case of Mrs. Jones whose diabetes is caused by obesity, sedentary lifestyle, not enough fiber and too much sugar and the wrong fats in her diet. All of these lifestyle factors team together to bring about insulin resistance, or Syndrome X. Mrs. Jones then develops Type 2 diabetes, which gives her fatigue, which furthers her junk food diet and sedentary lifestyle, which makes her diabetes worse, and on it goes. The hypoglycemic drugs that her doctors give her work briefly, then stop having any effect. The poor diet that Mrs. Jones is consuming is the "slamming the thumb in the desk drawer". Drs. A, B, and C are all working on a paradigm that they studied in medical school "if you can name it (the disease), then I can tame it (with drugs or surgery)". Medical approaches can be useful short term quick fixes to subdue symptoms, but do not address the crucial "slamming the thumb in the desk drawer". This book will.

DIABETES: SIMPLE BUT DEADLY.

At first glance, diabetes appears to be such a simple disease. Too much sugar in the blood. But that simple error creates an avalanche of problems in the body that create havoc with the health of diabetics, especially if they have poor regulation of their blood glucose. Diabetes is such an insidious disease that it is the leading cause of blindness, kidney disease, amputations, and heart disease in the US.[3]

And yet, if properly regulated, diabetes can become a minor limitation in life, which is how baseball legends Jackie Robinson and Catfish Hunter viewed their diabetes. Diabetes did not seriously curtail the accomplishments of diabetics Ray

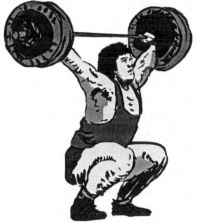

Kroc, multi-billionaire and founder of the MacDonald's empire; Hollywood celebrities Jack Benny, Mary Tyler Moore, and Ella Fitzgerald; U.S. Supreme Court Justice Oliver Wendell Holmes (who lived to age 94); and Ron Gillembardo, who at age 45 in 1992 in Barcelona became the oldest man in Olympic history to compete in powerlifting. Mr. Gillembardo told the press that, were it not for his diabetes and need to follow a strict diet, he could not have accomplished such an athletic feat at such an age.

Diabetes can become a wretched disease for those who ignore it, or an opportunity to make your life into a masterpiece for those who control it.

This book brings you a better understanding of this rampant disease, diabetes, and how to better control blood glucose levels using foods, supplements, and exercise. There is convincing evidence that you can improve quality and quantity of life and reduce complications for nearly all diabetics when using an aggressive nutrition program. Some Type 2 diabetics (non-insulin dependent) may actually have their disease go into complete remission by following the recommendations in this book. This book brings empowerment, therapeutic options, hope, wisdom, and a detailed game plan to you, the diabetic, to keep you out of harm's reach and filled with the zest of life.

INCIDENCE OF DIABETES IN US AND WORLD

In 1995, the National Institute of Diabetes and Digestive and Kidney Diseases estimated that 16 million Americans were suffering from some form of diabetes. Half of these people don't even know that they have the disease and may not receive adequate treatment until something serious happens, like blindness, kidney failure, heart attack, or gangrene sets in. In 1999, experts now estimate that 20 million Americans have diabetes with annual US health care costs at $105 billion.[4] Each day in America another 650,000 cases of diabetes are diagnosed. 120 million people around the globe suffer from diabetes. While 20% of Americans overall will develop diabetes in their lifetime, African Americans are twice as likely to develop diabetes compared to Anglos, and Latinos are even more prone toward diabetes than African Americans. All groups are at greater risk for developing diabetes as we age.

A LITTLE HISTORY ON DIABETES

Around 1500 BC, medical scribes in both India and Egypt described a condition of great thirst and urination. They treated this condition with high fiber wheat grain, a valid therapy which can be scientifically explained today. Over 3000 years ago, a treatment recommended for diabetes in India involved intensive exercise. Another ancient and good idea. It was the Greek Aretaeus around 100 AD who first called the disease "diabetes" after the Greek word for "siphon", noting all the excessive urination that diabetics experience.[5] Some of the earlier "medical technicians" would diagnose and track the severity of the diabetes based upon how sweet the patient's urine smelled. The more sugar in the urine, the more uncontrolled the disease and the greater the likelihood of suffering severe complications in the eyes, kidney, heart, and nerves. Thomas Willis, physician to King Charles II of England in 1670 was torn between commenting on the obvious increase in diabetes among his wealthy patrons eating lots of sugar and the wealth being made in the sugar trade by his boss.

In 1898, Elliott Joslin, MD emphasized the importance of diet, exercise, and lifestyle to control diabetes. Dr. Joslin's work became the foundation for the world famous Joslin Diabetes Center in Boston. Canadian researchers Frederick Banting and Charles Best first isolated insulin in 1921. Two years later, researchers Banting and Mcleod were awarded Nobel prizes for their work on insulin and diabetes. Demand for insulin was so high that a large pharmaceutical company, Eli Lilly, was required to meet the world's need for insulin. Since 1923, insulin research has brought various refinements, with the biggest breakthrough coming in 1978 when DNA engineering allowed researchers to manufacture human insulin, which has since become the gold standard for Type 1 insulin dependent diabetics.

In Joslin's era of 1898, the average life expectancy for a 10 year old diagnosed with Type 1 (insulin dependent) diabetes was 1.3 years. In the post-insulin era of 1945, that same 10 year old diabetic had a life expectancy of 45 years.[6] Even more progress has been made since then. But the experts all agree that the complications and life expectancy of the diabetic is directly related to how well blood glucose levels are regulated. This book will help greatly in that regulation.

CATEGORIES OF DIABETES

Let's make sure that we have the proper terminology for diabetes:

- ♥ Diabetes insipidus: disease of high urine output, possibly caused by lack of the pituitary hormone, anti-diuretic hormone.
- ♥ Diabetes mellitus: (means "siphoning sweetness") metabolic disease of too much glucose in the blood as caused by:

1) Lack of insulin output, type 1 diabetes, juvenile diabetic, Insulin Dependent Diabetes Mellitus (IDDM)

2) Ineffective insulin, meaning there is enough insulin but it does not effectively force glucose into the cells, type 2 diabetes, adult onset diabetes, Non Insulin Dependent Diabetes Mellitus (NIDDM)

Other forms of diabetes mellitus that are somewhat rare include:

-Secondary diabetes, which may be caused by pancreatic diseases, hormone disturbances, drug reactions, or malnutrition.

-Gestational diabetes, which is glucose intolerance brought on during pregnancy.

Only 5% of diabetics qualify as Type 1, which is caused by destruction of the insulin-producing cells of the pancreas (beta cells). Some possible causes of the beta cell destruction include an auto-immune attack (the body's own immune system ganging up on the pancreas) triggered by a food allergy, especially from milk. Infants under 4 months of age who were fed cow's milk have a 50% greater risk of developing Type 1 diabetes than infants who are breastfed. When diabetes is in the family, cow's milk may need to be avoided in newborn infants.

The remaining 90%+ of all diabetics are Type 2, non insulin dependent. And 90% of these diabetics are overweight, which is a huge risk factor for diabetes. We will talk more about this later. While all diabetics can glean some valuable information from this book, the focus of this book is for Type 2 diabetics. All diabetics need to continue working with your physician while incorporating the recommendations from this book into your lifestyle.

CAN MY DOCTOR CURE DIABETES?

No. Diabetes has become so common that Americans spend $12 billion annually on research and $105 billion on therapy. This monumental effort has allowed medical science

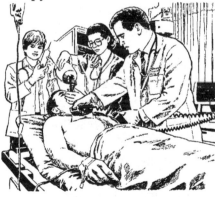 to better manage the secondary diseases of diabetes. But slowing the consequences is very different from curing the disease. Routine medical therapy would consist of the following:

Type 1 diabetic. Intensified insulin therapy, which is designed to mimic the flow of insulin in a healthy human. 3-5 injections of human insulin (or flow from an attached pump) are spaced throughout the day in accordance with meals. Outcome with Type 1 diabetes is vastly superior than even a few decades ago. Yet, the American Diabetic Association admits that it is a rare Type 1 diabetic who will live 50 years with the disease. In Britain prior to the discovery of insulin (1922), there were 119 deaths from diabetes per million people. After the discovery of insulin (1931) there were 145 deaths from diabetes per million population. Clearly, insulin helps control the rampant complications from diabetes, but is far from a cure for the disease.

Type 2 diabetic. Use of oral hypoglycemic agents, including sulfa drugs like Diabinese, Glucotrol, Micronase, and Orinase. These drugs seem to enhance insulin production and the sensitivity of the body cells to insulin. However, they lose their effectiveness with time and, according to a huge study by the University Group Diabetes Program, elevate the risk for death from heart attack or stroke by 250%.[7] Other treatment drugs include metformin, the thiazolidinediones (TZDs), insulin, acarbose (blocks starch digestion), and orlistat (blocks fat digestion). All of these drugs have their considerable side effects, such as orlistat, which causes flatulence, oily stools, "rectal leakage", and malabsorption of the fat soluble vitamins A, D, E, and K.[8]

WHAT ARE THE COMPLICATIONS OF DIABETES?

Remember, this is a loaded question. The statistics regarding diabetics in America are not very encouraging. However, the diseases that affect the diabetic are started and exaggerated by poor blood glucose control. You can minimize your risk for the following conditions. But be aware that ignoring your diabetes puts you in a high risk category for problems of the:

♥ Circulatory system, including heart disease, stroke, poor circulation to the feet and hands. 80% of Type 2 diabetics die from heart disease.

♥ Shriveling of the tiny blood vessels leading to problems in the eyes, a.k.a. retinopathy. 15 years after diagnosis, 90%

of Type 1 and 80% of Type 2 diabetics show some damage to the retina of the eyes.

♥ Kidney complications, or nephropathy. The vast majority of American patients on renal dialysis are diabetics.

♥ Nerve damage, or neuropathy, leading to tingling, painful, "pins & needles" sensations in the hands and feet.

♥ Nerve damage to the bladder, intestines, sexual organs, etc. and the consequences of losing the contributions from those organs or regions of the body.

♥ Ulcers of the leg and foot, which are combined problems of nerves and blood vessels.

WILL THIS PROGRAM IMPROVE MY TYPE 2 DIABETES?

Yes. Since 90% of Type 2 diabetics are obese, weight reduction can dramatically improve blood glucose regulation and even cure the diabetes.[9] Obesity may distort the "landing sites" for insulin on the cell membrane, not unlike blowing up a balloon larger than normal and watching the writing on the balloon become distorted. There is reason to believe that many people can dramatically improve blood glucose regulation merely by eating a "hunter gatherer diet" consisting of lean and clean meat (chicken, turkey, fish, lean beef and pork) along with complex carbohydrates rich in soluble fiber (vegetables, whole grains, nuts, seeds, fruit, legumes).

Researcher Dr. O'Dea in Australia wondered if the modern refined diet of many Aborigines living in Sidney, Australia could cause diabetes. He recruited 10 full blooded male aborigines who had Type 2 diabetes and asked them to return to the "hunter gatherer" diet of their ancestors. All 10 subjects were middle age and overweight. Seven weeks after beginning their ancestral diet, all 10 men had lost an average of 16 pounds in spite of making no effort to reduce weight, all had experienced a 50% drop in blood lipids (lowering their risk for heart disease), and all had such splendid improvement in fasting blood glucose levels that they were considered "cured" of Type 2 diabetes.[10]

Max Gerson, MD was a well-respected German neurosurgeon in the 1920s. He began treating "refractory" diseases of all sorts, including diabetes, lupus, and cancer with a basic program of nutrition and detoxification. Dr. Gerson used his simple program to cure the wife of the famous medical missionary, Dr. Albert Schweitzer, from advanced tuberculosis in 1928, and then cured Schweitzer himself of Type 2 diabetes, allowing Schweitzer to live another 15 years to age 90.[11]

BLOOD SUGAR, FOOD SUGAR, AND THE DISEASES OF CIVILIZATION

In the 1930s, a dentist Weston Price, and his wife/nurse, decided to quit their practices and travel the world in the ultimate "Indiana Jones" scientific study and adventure. Travelling on propellar planes to 12 cultures on 5 continents, they found that people who consumed their ancestral diet had both good teeth and generally good health. Once these people adopted the "western diet" (Read: refined carbohydrates lacking in fiber) then both the teeth and general health of these varied cultures began to rapidly deteriorate.[12] Diabetes was virtually never seen in people who followed their native ethnic diet.

Drs. Shostak, Eaton, and Konner of Emory University studied the lifestyle of the few remaining "hunter gatherer" cultures around the world and compared their diet to ours, then published this research in the prestigious New England Journal of Medicine and as a book, THE PALEOLITHIC PRESCRIPTION. There is a huge gap between what we modern Americans are currently eating and what our bodies are designed to require.[13] Note the following chart which shows that we Americans get 19% of our calories from simple carbohydrates, mostly white sugar. Our ancestors got almost no calories from simple carbohydrates, except for the brief harvest time for fruits in the summer and fall. The glycemic index of real fruit usually is much better than the glycemic index of refined sugars. Glycemic index basically tells us how fast the sugar gets into our bloodstream. More on the importance of the glycemic index later.

TIME RELEASE FOOD SUPPLY

For thousands of years, our ancestors ate foods that slowly released their calories in the process of digestion, to be eventually absorbed into the bloodstream and easily handled by a meager supply of insulin. However, modern Americans have ignored this biological adaptation of our bodies and consume huge amounts of refined carbohydrates to bring about a rush of easily absorbed sugars into the bloodstream.

Fiber in whole foods slows down the absorption of sugar into the bloodstream so that blood glucose stays at a manageable level. With the 140 pounds per year of refined white sugar consumed annually by the average American, and the fact that the most commonly eaten food in America is white bread, we now literally inject sugars into our bloodstream. This is one of the main reasons for the epidemic proportions of diabetes in America.

Diabetes is one of the more prevalent, lethal, expensive, and easily reversed conditions in America. The vast majority of diabetes is caused by ignoring the basic laws of Nature. Humans need "time release" foods that slowly allow small amounts of carbohydrates to be absorbed into the bloodstream. We are built for activity and get sick when we overeat or develop obesity. 95% of all sugar in the blood is supposed to be burned by the muscles, yet sedentary Americans end up having that sugar linger in the blood until the insulin supply can force the sugar either into storage as glycogen or storage as fat. We have a nutritional need for a wide assortment of nutrients involved in burning sugar in our cell furnaces, not unlike needing spark plugs in your car to burn the gasoline in your engine. These "spark plugs" that are deficient in our Standard American Diet (SAD) include magnesium, chromium, vanadium, and omega-3 fats from fish and flax oils.

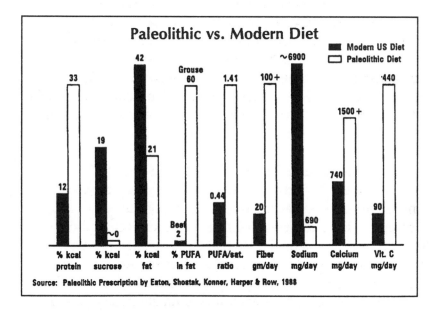

Most of our hunter-gatherer ancestors ate a diet consisting of about 1/3 lean animal tissue with the remaining 2/3 of the diet unprocessed plant food; mostly vegetables, some grains, some fruit, nuts, seeds and legumes. If the creature runs, flies, or swims, then it may be about 4% body fat, with obvious exceptions including duck and salmon. Cows, the staple meat of America, do not run, swim, or fly and are about

30-40% body fat after they have been fattened at the feedlot with hormones, corn meal and the inability to move. The basic diet of our ancestors that will help you control your diabetes is lean and clean protein foods along with complex carbohydrates in their natural state.

Keep in mind that you may have to "fine tune" this paleolithic diet to suit your ethnic background. The macrobiotic diet was developed by a Japanese physician who cured himself of cancer in the 19th century. The macrobiotic diet tends to encourage anything Oriental, even soy sauce and pickles, and discourage anything Western, including chicken, turkey, fish and fruit. Macrobiotics may be ideally suited for many Orientals, and has helped some Caucasians because it is such a vast improvement over the nutritional quality of the typical American diet. I encourage people to determine the diet of their ancestors 1000 years ago and use that food pattern as a starting point.

WHAT ARE THE "ROOTS" OF DIABETES?

Anthropologists (scientists who study the origins of humans) tell us that humans were originally "hunters and gatherers". Then came the Ice Age, in which vast regions of the earth were covered with ice and the remaining parts of the earth were much colder than normal. This Ice Age, obviously, was not conducive to farming and the availability of lots of plant food. So most of our ancestors, until about 25,000 years ago when the ice began receding to its current position, were meat eaters. Meanwhile, glucose, which only comes from plant food, is the most essential fuel in the human body. The brain, lens of the eye, lungs, and kidneys must have glucose to operate properly. The brain is so dependent on glucose that it does not even need insulin to get glucose into the cells, which is unusual, since nearly all other body cells require insulin and the Glucose Tolerance Factor (GTF) to enable glucose to slip in through the cell membrane.

Back to our ancient ancestors. They consumed very little carbohydrates, and what little they consumed had to be quickly shuttled to the cells for fuel, lest the glucose linger in the bloodstream and cause some damage. People who did not eat much plant food, such as those groups from the colder climates in northern Europe, developed an ability to make glucose from the proteins in our diet (called gluconeogenesis). As you will see in upcoming chapters, glucose is sort of a necessary evil for body cells. If just the right amount of glucose goes straight from the intestinal absorption to the body cells and is burned for fuel, then the person feels great and lives a long and healthy life. If too little glucose is available, then the person feels cranky, depressed, forgetful and listless in the condition called hypoglycemia (low sugar levels in the blood). If an excess of glucose starts accumulating outside of the cell, then "glucotoxicity" begins. Glucotoxicity is a slow but lethal process whereby too much glucose outside of the cells triggers a host of destructive pathways throughout the body.

Once farming began, around 8000 years ago in the Middle East, then our ancestors found the ability to settle down, start cities, and begin the processes of civilization. Then, around 1600 AD, came the refining of wheat in northern Europe. This new technique allowed the wheat miller to strip the outer bran and inner germ from the whole wheat kernel for a fine "Queen's white" flour. Around 1700 AD, trade ships would run the triangle of taking African slaves to the Carribean, where the ships would pick up cane sugar, molasses, and rum from the southern plantations and bring these products to Europe. Once refined cane sugar was brought to the masses, the health of millions began to deteriorate rapidly. Enter the dawning of the "diseases of civilization", especially diabetes.

Based upon hundreds of scientific studies, Type 2 diabetes is well recognized as a disease that is a consequence of our modern lifestyle:

♥ obesity
♥ too much refined carbohydrates with too little fiber to slow down the absorption of the sugar
♥ sedentary lifestyle
♥ too little minerals (like chromium, magnesium, and vanadium) in our diet due to the negligence of agribusiness
♥ too much fat and the wrong kind of fat in our diet which leads to changes in cell membranes that no longer recognize the role of insulin.

You will learn more about all of these lifestyle factors later. Basically, the bad news is that diabetes is at epidemic

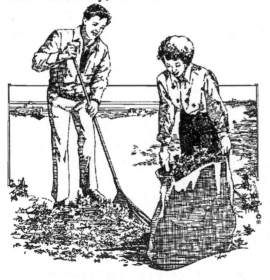

proportions in America and getting worse. The good news is that diabetes is lifestyle induced and lifestyle controlled. How much diabetes will influence your quality and quantity of life will largely depend on you. You are to be congratulated for purchasing this book. You will reap a thousand fold benefits when you begin to implement these recommendations in your daily living.

PATIENT PROFILE

D.M. was a colleague of mine at work who had developed fatigue, frequency of urination, and thirst all of which just didn't seem right. At age 44 and overweight, her doctor suspected diabetes. And, unfortunately, her doctor was right. D.M. has just joined the 20 million Americans with diabetes, a disease that has been relatively rare until this century. She ignored her diabetes for a year before she came to me for help. She started a diet that is outlined in this book, with particular emphasis on the superfoods. She began taking nutrition supplements, including chromium and the herb Gymnema. Within 2 months on this program, she called me one Saturday morning to tell me how much more alive she felt and how her cuts and scratches were healing much quicker.

ENDNOTES

[1]. Bennett, PH, Nutr.Rev., vol.57, no.5, p.S51, 1999

[2]. Cohen, AM, et al., Lancet, vol.2, p.1399, 1961

[3]. Drum, D., et al., TYPE II DIABETES SOURCEBOOK, p.6, Lowell House, Los Angeles, 1998

[4]. Rubin, RJ, et al., J.Clin.Endocrin.Metab., vol.78, p.809A, 1994

[5]. Mitchell, J. (ed), RANDOM HOUSE ENCYCLOPEDIA, p.726, Random House, NY, 1983

[6]. Thomas, M., et al., THE UNOFFICIAL GUIDE TO LIVING WITH DIABETES, p.413, Macmillan, NY, 1999

[7]. UDGP, Diabetes, vol.19, p.789, 1970

[8]. Halstead, CH, Am.J.Clin.Nutr., vol.69, p.1059, 1999

[9]. Campbell, PJ, et al., Diabetes, vol.42, p.405, 1993

[10]. O'Dea, K., Diabetes, vol.33, p.596, June 1984

[11]. Schmid, RF, NATIVE NUTRITION, p.89, Healing Arts Press, Rochester, VT, 1994

[12]. Price, WA, NUTRITION AND PHYSICAL DEGENERATION, Keats, New Canaan, CT, 1945

[13]. Eaton, SB, et al., New England Journal of Medicine, vol.312, no.5, p.283, Jan.1985

CHAPTER 2

KILLING US SWEETLY
EXCESS SUGAR AS A WRECKING
BALL IN THE BODY

"If you find honey, eat just enough--too much of it, and you will vomit." Proverbs 25:16

This chapter is included not to scare you, but to convince you of the urgency in controlling your blood glucose.

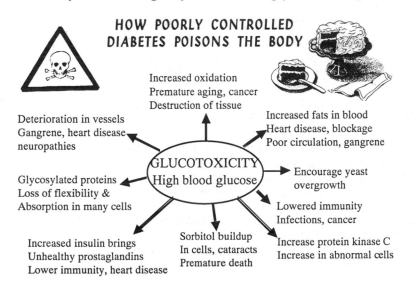

HOW POORLY CONTROLLED DIABETES POISONS THE BODY

Increased oxidation
Premature aging, cancer
Destruction of tissue

Deterioration in vessels
Gangrene, heart disease
neuropathies

Increased fats in blood
Heart disease, blockage
Poor circulation, gangrene

GLUCOTOXICITY
High blood glucose

Glycosylated proteins
Loss of flexibility &
Absorption in many cells

Encourage yeast
overgrowth

Lowered immunity
Infections, cancer

Increased insulin brings
Unhealthy prostaglandins
Lower immunity, heart disease

Sorbitol buildup
In cells, cataracts
Premature death

Increase protein kinase C
Increase in abnormal cells

Half of the 20 million Americans with diabetes don't know or don't care about the disease. Many diabetics will ignore doctor and nutritionist recommendations because these lifestyle changes seem inconvenient. While high blood sugar does not hurt anyone in the beginning, it initiates an avalanche of biological problems that cannot be stopped by any drug or nutrient.

DIFFERENCES in ENERGY METABOLISM BETWEEN NORMAL & DIABETIC CELLS

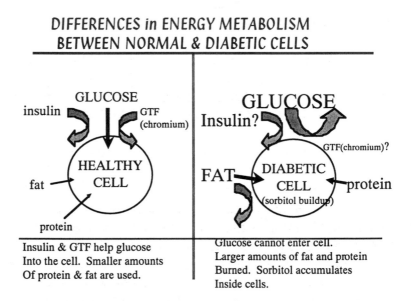

| Insulin & GTF help glucose Into the cell. Smaller amounts Of protein & fat are used. | Glucose cannot enter cell. Larger amounts of fat and protein Burned. Sorbitol accumulates Inside cells. |

While we have known for centuries that poorly controlled diabetes leads to many complications, it was not until recently that scientists could explain how excess glucose poisons the system. Excess blood glucose accumulates outside of the cell. The free glucose begins to attach to various blood proteins in the process of glycosylation...essentially "tanning" these cell membranes and various proteins to reduce their flexibility and absorption properties. Meanwhile the cell inside is starving for fuel. So the cell begins to burn fat, but rather inefficiently, leading to higher blood fats circulating through the 60,000 miles of blood vessels. The residue particles of incomplete combustion of fats are called ketone bodies and leave the diabetic with breath like an alcoholic, some confusion, and often a sense of "who cares" about this condition.

Excess sugar in the blood begins a rapid acceleration of the oxidation, or wearing out, of all cells. This oxidation increases the aging process, rusting the nerves to bring neuropathies (or tingling and painful nerves), shriveling the blood vessels in the eyes for possible blindness, starving the kidneys for possible renal failure, and shutting down circulation to the distant extremities for possible gangrene. Excess blood glucose lets a monster out of the bag: protein kinase C, which generates too much cell division, possibly leading to cancer.

It has been well documented that cancer is a "sugar feeder", or an obligate glucose utilizer.[1] There is a direct relationship between countries that eat the most sugar and the incidence of breast cancer. Also, insulin is a powerful growth (anabolic) hormone which can accelerate cancer spread.[2] When the diabetic cannot use or even store the excess blood sugar, opportunistic yeast living in all of us can readily start growing on the sugar and leave the diabetic with a systemic yeast infection, which starts another cascade of health problems.

Excess insulin from insulin resistance, Type 2 diabetes, then starts another cascade of events by switching a "Y" fork in metabolism to make more unfriendly prostaglandin PGE-2, which causes constriction of blood vessels, lowering immunity, increasing the stickiness of all cells (greater risk for heart disease, stroke, and the spreading of cancer), and more. All these problems stem from something as simple as too much sugar in the blood, or what scientists now call "glucotoxicity".[3]

HOW IS BLOOD GLUCOSE MEASURED?

In order to be diagnosed with diabetes, most clinicians will rely on the oral glucose tolerance test, or OGTT. In this

ORAL GLUCOSE TOLERANCE TEST
MONITORING BLOOD GLUCOSE LEVELS

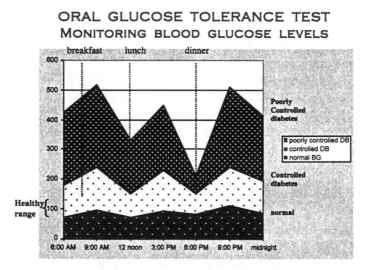

test, the patient shows up at the clinic in the morning after a 12 hour fast. A blood sample is drawn, then a glass of sweet fluid (glucose solution) is consumed by the patient. Then blood samples are drawn every 30-60 minutes for the next 3-6 hours. This OGTT allows the doctor to determine how rapidly the body absorbs glucose and how quickly insulin is produced and able to force the blood glucose into the cells. Blood glucose levels are judged by:

60-110 milligrams per deciliter of blood (mg%)=normal
below 60 mg%=hypoglycemia
above 126 mg%=possible diabetes

Essentially, the diabetic is trying to take the "highs and lows" out of the swings in blood glucose. This is easier said than done. But the foods and supplements discussed later can make this smoothing out of the blood glucose extremes quite possible.

INSULIN RESISTANCE

In 1988, a well respected physician researcher, Dr. Gerald Reaven, of Stanford University Medical Center published his findings on this growing problem of insulin resistance, or Syndrome X.[4] Essentially, a large and growing percentage (25% by Reaven's estimate) of the "healthy" non-obese non-diabetic population in the US are suffering from insulin resistance, which means that the body makes enough insulin, but the insulin cannot seem to "open the door" of the cell membrane to allow glucose to enter the cell. Insulin resistance is a leading cause of Type 2 diabetes, along with rises in hypertension (over 60 million Americans have high blood pressure), and heart disease (still the leading cause of death in the US).

The cell membrane receptor for insulin could be compared to the uniqueness of a fingerprint. This receptor is a 3 dimensional site on the cell membrane that must be in proper working order for insulin to do its job. Realize that the average healthy non-diabetic individual secretes around 31 units of insulin daily, while the Type 2 obese diabetic secretes 114 units daily!!! This is nearly 4 times the normal amount. Lean Type 2 diabetics, which are rare, secrete 14 units of insulin daily and Type 1 insulin dependent diabetics make an average of 4 units of insulin each day.[5]

The reason that too much insulin is made and still doesn't do the job is the improper structure from the wrong building materials for the insulin receptors on the cell membrane. This "gatekeeper" of the cell is composed of a fatty (lipid) layer of very specific fats. But Americans feed ourselves the wrong kind of fats (hydrogenated, saturated) which become incorporated into the cell membrane and not enough of the right kinds of fats (EPA and DHA from fish, ALA from flax, GLA from borage and primrose) along with deficiencies of minerals like magnesium, sulfur, chromium, and vanadium that assist in this crucial insulin receptor site on the cell membrane. More on this subject, including how to fix the problem, when we get to the chapters on superfoods, nutritious & delicious, and nutritional supplements.

PATIENT PROFILE

S.R. was a retired widow looking forward to travel and enjoying her grandkids when the doctor diagnosed her with Type 2 diabetes. She came to me with a determination to enjoy her golden years and do whatever it takes to beat her diabetes. I suggested a flax oil salad dressing to replace her favorite blue cheese dressing. She joined the local YWCA and became an enthusiast of calisthenics in the swimming pool. With the addition of brewer's yeast and other nutrition supplements, she was able to discontinue her medication and spent the next 5 years in vigorous pursuit of exotic travel and her grandkids. For S.R., the diagnosis of "diabetes" was merely a wakeup call to get started on her long overdue fitness program, which gave her more energy than she had had in decades.

ENDNOTES

[1]. Rothkopf, M., Nutrition, vol.6, no.4, p.14S, July/Aug.1990 supplement

[2]. Yam, D., Medical Hypotheses, vol.38, p.111, 1992

[3]. Mooradian, AD, et al., Advances in Care of Older People w.Diabetes, vol.15, no.2, p.255, May 1999

[4]. Reaven, GM, Diabetes, vol.37, p.1595, Dec.1988

[5]. Murray, M., ENCYCLOPEDIA OF NATURAL MEDICINE, p.409, Prima Publ, 1998

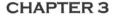

CHAPTER 3

GLYCEMIC INDEX

HOW QUICK DOES THE FOOD SUGAR GET INTO THE BLOODSTREAM?

"Almost every second store and shop in our villages and cities is a candy store, and common sense and common observation knows well enough the morbid results. How many patients have blessed me for the suggestion to stop all sweets and have traced to the continued rules their reinstated health and enjoyment of life." Dr. George M. Gould, physician in 1910

Humans are not built to withstand the rigors of many aspects of modern life. We are going deaf at an alarming rate due to noise pollution and prematurely hardened arteries in the ear region. Our ancestors had reasonably good hearing throughout their long and productive lives. In primitive societies, people in their 70s have hearing better than many of our teenagers in America, due to avoidance of noise pollution.

The same thing is happening with respect to sugar, refined carbohydrates, and fiber-depleted foods in America. Our bodies are not built to withstand the constant flood of simple sugars entering our bloodstream. If we were active and burning up the sugar in work, then the sugar would be of less consequence. But we sip and munch on sweet foods all day long while sitting at our desks or in front of the TV, then wonder why morbid obesity has increased by 300% since the introduction of aspartame, the artificial sweetener.

Earlier nutritionists simply said, "Stop eating all sweet food!" to their diabetic patients. This is easier said than done, when many diabetics have become "sugar addicts". A more exacting scientific approach to the role of dietary carbohydrates in blood glucose levels was developed in 1981 by Dr. David Jenkins. While some health care professionals consider the glycemic index the "gold standard" in guiding diabetic patients, I consider it one of many guidelines that are important. For example, spaghetti and Uncle Ben's white rice, which are highly refined foods, appear to have a more favorable glycemic index (GI) than buckwheat groats or beets, which are whole foods. Yet buckwheat is rich in magnesium, fiber, vitamin E and other nutrients found in whole grains. Beets are a treasure trove of phytochemicals, or chemicals in plants that protect us from various diseases and premature aging. Meanwhile, white flour spaghetti noodles and white rice have had at least 24 nutrients removed and 4 added back. This nutritional robbery occurs daily in the American food supply and needs to be taken into consideration when using the GI to make dietary recommendations.

Another issue is that GI may seem to favor white sugar, or sucrose, over whole grain bread. Yet, when an equal amount of calories from either sucrose or wheat starch were fed to animals, the sucrose diet yielded more than a 50% increase in the number of tumors.[1] In other words, refined simple carbohydrates need to be seriously limited, even if we cannot explain that limitation based on glycemic index alone.

With that caveat in mind, let's explain how the GI was developed and what it means to you, the diabetic reader. Human subjects, both healthy and diabetic, are fed 50 grams of carbohydrates from various foods. For instance, people are fed

200 grams of spaghetti in order to get 50 grams of carbohydrates, because spaghetti also contains some protein, fat, water, and fiber. Researchers then compare the size of the Oral Glucose Tolerance Test curve. If a food creates only half the rise in blood glucose compared to consuming a pure glucose drink, then the food gets a GI rating of 50, and so on.

The more that you process a food, the higher the GI becomes. Cooked whole wheat berries have a GI of 41, white bread has a GI of 70. The more the food is stripped of its fiber and ground into smaller particles, the higher the GI and the worse that food becomes for the diabetic.

You might say that ice cream has a better GI than whole wheat bread, so eat more ice cream?? Actually, the sugar and fat in ice cream are likely to make the diabetic risks for heart disease even more prominent. Use this glycemic index table[2] as it was meant to be used: As a guideline to help people make the right food choices, not as the only nutrition tool for good judgment at the dinner table.

PATIENT PROFILE

T.B. was a very successful businessman who was told that he was diabetic on his 50th birthday. He took the usual approach,"Get me an expert on this subject!! I've got good insurance." He took his medication, but ignored my advice regarding diet and supplements and generally did not take good care of himself. He died 3 years later of a heart attack.

ENDNOTES

[1]. Hoehn, SK, et al., Nutrition and Cancer, vol.1, no.3, p.27, 1983

[2]. Brand-Miller, J., et al., THE GLUCOSE REVOLUTION, Marlowe, NYC, 1999

GLYCEMIC INDEX:

how fast does the carbohydrate food get into the blood compared to glucose (=100)

	bread/grain	vegetables	fruit	legumes	dairy	beverages	snack food
90-100		parsnip, baked white potato	dried dates (103)				glucose, maltose (105)
80-89	corn flakes, crispbread,	red skinned potato					
70-79	raisin bran, vanilla wafers, graham crackers, waffles, white & wheat bread, bagel, cocoa krispies	french fries, pumpkin	watermelon	broad beans		Gatorade	corn chips, Life Savers, Skittles Fruit Chews,
60-69	taco shells, shredded wheat, arrowroot cookies, shortbread,	beets, new potatoes	cantaloupe, pineapple, raisins		ice cream	soft drink syrup, Fanta	sucrose (white sugar), Mars almond bar,
50-59	all bran, stone ground whole wheat, buckwheat, brown & white rice, blueberry muffin, pita & sourdough bread,	sweet corn, sweet potato, yam	banana, kiwi, mango, papaya				Power bar, potato chips, honey, popcorn
40-49	noodles, sponge cake, spachetti, oatmeal, banana bread,	carrots, green peas,	grapes, orange,	baked beans		orange juice, apple juice,	chocolate, Twix Cookie Snickers, lactose
30-39	pasta fettuccine, ravioli,		apple, apricot, pear, plum	butter beans, chick peas (garbanzo), lentils, navy beans	low fat yogurt, skim milk, chocolate milk		
20-29			cherries, grapefruit	kidney beans	whole milk		fructose
10-19				soybeans			peanuts

CHAPTER 4

MALNUTRITION IN AMERICA

NUTRITION SURVIVAL FACTS

"Our way of life is related to our way of death." the Framingham study, Harvard University

Most Americans know more facts about their favorite baseball team than basic facts on nutrition. Most Americans "live to eat", but fail to realize that all forms of life on earth must "eat to live". Understanding some basics about nutrition and the nutritionally bankrupt food that permeates our American diet is crucial for you, the diabetic reader, to start a healthier lifestyle.

Howard Hughes, the multi-billionaire, died of malnutrition. It is hard to believe that there can be malnutrition in this agriculturally abundant nation of ours--but there is. At the time of the Revolutionary War, 96% of Americans farmed while only 4% worked at other trades. Tractors and harvesting combines became part of an agricultural revolution that allowed the 2% of Americans who now farm to feed the rest of us. We grow enough food in this country to feed ourselves, to make half of us overweight, to throw away enough food to feed 50 million people daily, to ship food overseas as a major export, and to store enough food in government surplus bins to feed Americans for a year if all farmers quit today. With so much food available, how can Americans be malnourished?

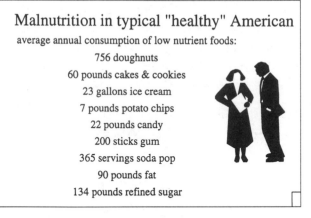

Malnutrition in typical "healthy" American

average annual consumption of low nutrient foods:

756 doughnuts

60 pounds cakes & cookies

23 gallons ice cream

7 pounds potato chips

22 pounds candy

200 sticks gum

365 servings soda pop

90 pounds fat

134 pounds refined sugar

The answer is: poor food choices. Americans chose their food based upon taste, cost, convenience and psychological gratification--thus ignoring the main reason that we eat, which is to provide our body cells with the raw materials to grow, repair and fuel our bodies. The most commonly eaten foods in America are white bread, coffee and hot dogs. Based upon our food abundance, Americans could be the best nourished nation on record. But we are far from it.

CAUSES OF NUTRIENT DEFICIENCIES

⇒ Don't eat it.

⇒ Don't absorb it.

⇒ Don't keep it. Increased excretion or loss of nutrients can be due to diarrhea, vomiting or drug interactions.

⇒ Don't get enough. Increased nutrient requirements can be due to fever, disease (like diabetes), alcohol or drug interactions.

Are you confused about why we Americans spend $1.5
trillion per year on medical care, more than any other nation in
history, and another $12 billion at the National Institutes of
Health for research and then somehow have twice the incidence
of diabetes compared to ten years ago?   You might be
surprised at what sells best in American grocery stores.

Overwhelming evidence from both government and

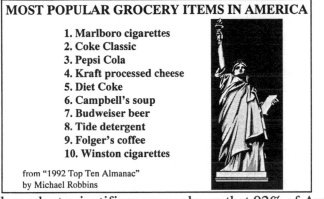

MOST POPULAR GROCERY ITEMS IN AMERICA

1. **Marlboro cigarettes**
2. **Coke Classic**
3. **Pepsi Cola**
4. **Kraft processed cheese**
5. **Diet Coke**
6. **Campbell's soup**
7. **Budweiser beer**
8. **Tide detergent**
9. **Folger's coffee**
10. **Winston cigarettes**

from "1992 Top Ten Almanac"
by Michael Robbins

independent scientific surveys shows that 92% of Americans
do not get the Recommended Dietary Allowance for all
essential nutrients. Specifically, we are low in our intake of:[1]

VITAMINS: A, D, E, C, B-6, riboflavin, folacin, pantothenate
MINERALS: calcium, potassium, magnesium, zinc, iron,
chromium, selenium; and possibly molybdenum and vanadium.
MACRONUTRIENTS: fiber, complex carbohydrates, plant
protein, special fatty acids (EPA, GLA, ALA), clean water

Meanwhile, we also eat alarmingly high amounts of:
fat, salt, sugar, cholesterol, alcohol, caffeine, food additives and
toxins.

This combination of too much of the wrong things
along with not enough of the right things has created epidemic
proportions of degenerative diseases in this country, including

diabetes. The Surgeon General, Department of Health and Human Services, Center for Disease Control, National Academy of Sciences, American Medical Association, American Dietetic Assocation, and most other major public health agencies agree that diet is a major contributor to our most common health problems. Even the conservative report from the Surgeon General states: "Some estimates suggest that new cases of diabetes could be reduced by nearly half by preventing obesity in middle-aged adults."[2]

The typical diet of the diabetic patient is high in fat while being low in fiber and vegetables--"meat, potatoes, and gravy" is what many of my patients lived on. Data collected by the United States Department of Agriculture from over 11,000 Americans showed that on any given day:

♥ 41 percent did not eat any fruit
♥ 82 percent did not eat cruciferous vegetables
♥ 72 percent did not eat vitamin C-rich fruits or vegetables
♥ 80 percent did not eat vitamin A-rich fruits or vegetables
♥ 84 percent did not eat high fiber grain food, like bread or cereal[3]

The human body is incredibly resilient, which sometimes works to our disadvantage. No one dies on the first cigarette inhaled, or the first drunken evening, or the first decade of unhealthy eating. We misconstrue the fact that we survived this ordeal to mean we can do it forever. Not so. Malnutrition can be blatant, as the starving babies in third world countries. Malnutrition can also be much more subtle.

MACRONUTRIENTS: We eat protein, carbohydrates, and fats in large quantities, hence they are sometimes referred to as macronutrients (meaning "big" nutrients). We also eat fiber, which is indigestible parts of plant foods. Since fiber is indigestible and therefore cannot enter the bloodstream, scientists assumed back in the 1950s that fiber was useless and stripping it from the food supply was totally acceptable. Bad idea. Logic would assume that something found in our food supply for thousands of years must have a purpose. Yet, it was not until the 1970s that a British physician, Dennis Burkitt, working in Africa noticed an entirely different set of diseases among Africans who ate a high fiber diet compared to Europeans and Americans who eat a highly refined low-fiber diet.

Fiber may be one of the more important elements in your diabetes recovery program. Fiber binds up toxins and fat in the intestines, carrying them out with the feces. Fiber slows down the absorption of carbohydrates and improves the glycemic index of foods. Soluble fiber, such as found in many vegetables, oat bran, sea vegetables, legumes, and other foods will be outlined in the "superfoods" section later on.

MICRONUTRIENTS. We consume vitamins (like C, E, A, D, and the B vitamins) and minerals (like selenium, chromium, and magnesium) in smaller quantities, hence the name "micro", meaning small.

The reason I bring up these basic nutrition facts is that many Americans are suffering from long term subclinical deficiencies of various nutrients that can induce or worsen diabetes. In the chapter on "nutrition supplements that may be of benefit" you will learn about vitamins, minerals, herbs, food extracts, and fatty acids that may dramatically improve the course of health for the diabetic. You might ask: "Why do I need these nutrients now? If I have been low in my intake of them all along, then why didn't I get sick earlier?"

In the hierarchy of nutrient needs, we must have oxygen

NUTRITIONAL DEFICIENCIES

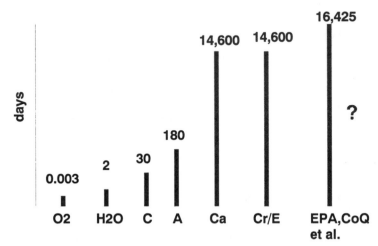

first; because 5 minutes without oxygen and we are dead. Next
in line is water. We can last a couple of days without water.
Next is calories, since we can live for 2 months or more
without any food intake, other than water. Next are the
micronutrients of vitamins and minerals. It might take 20 years
of low intake of calcium to bring about osteoporosis, or
hollowing of the bones. It might take 20-40 years of low intake
of vitamin E to bring about excess rusting of fats in the
bloodstream and a fatal heart attack. These nutrient
deficiencies do not surface quickly, but they are important in
the long run. Surviving does not equal thriving. We may be
able to survive for decades without optimal amounts of
chromium in the diet, but we become a ticking time bomb
waiting for some health disaster to occur. More on this subject

when we talk about nutrition supplements in an upcoming chapter.

Many diabetics suffer from long term low intake of a wide assortment of nutrients. In some cases, diabetics need more than the average healthy person, as in the case of vitamin C. In some cases, few Americans get enough of these nutrients, such as chromium, magnesium, or fish oil.

This chapter was included to provide you with some basic facts regarding common malnutrition in the "healthy" American, and even more common malnutrition in the "well controlled" diabetic, which then leads to many nasty complications. We are going to make sure that you are optimally nourished, which will dramatically improve the course of your diabetes.

The KISS (keep it simple, student) method of optimal nutrition.

✓ Go natural. Eat foods in as close to their natural state as possible. Refining food often adds questionable agents (like food additives, salt, sugar and fat), removes valuable nutrients (like vitamins, minerals, and fiber) and always raises the cost of the food.

✓ Expand your horizons. Eat a wide variety of foods. By not focusing on any particular food, you can obtain nutrients that may be essential but are poorly understood while also avoiding a buildup of any substance that could create food allergies or toxicities.

✓ Nibbling is better. Eat small frequent meals. Nibbling is better than gorging. Our ancestors "grazed" throughout the day. Only with the advent of the industrial age did we begin the punctual eating of large meals. Nibbling helps to stabilize blood sugar levels and minimize insulin rushes; therefore has been linked to a lowered risk for heart disease, diabetes, obesity and mood swings.

✓ Avoid problem foods. Minimize your intake of unhealthy foods which are high in fat, salt, sugar, cholesterol, caffeine, alcohol, processed lunch meats and most additives.

✓ Seek out nutrient-dense foods. Maximize your intake of life-giving foods, including fresh vegetables, whole grains, legumes, fruit, low fat meat (turkey, fish, chicken) and clean water. Low fat dairy products, especially yogurt, can be valuable if you do not have milk allergies or lactose intolerance.

✓ Monitor your quality of weight, rather than quantity of weight. Balance your calorie intake with expenditure so that your percentage of body fat is reasonable. Pinch the skinfold just above the hipbone. If this skin is more than an inch in thickness, then you may need to begin rational efforts to lose weight. Obesity is a major factor in diabetes. How much you weigh is not nearly as crucial as the percent of fat in the body. Skinfold thickness above the hipbone is a decent way of monitoring your percent body fat.

✓ Eat enough protein. Take in 1 to 2 grams of protein for each kilogram of body weight. Example: 150 pound patient. Divide 150 pounds by 2.2 to find 68 kilograms, multiply times 1 to 2, yields 68 to 136 grams of protein daily is needed.

✓ Use supplements in addition to, rather than instead of, good food. Get your nutrients with a fork and spoon. Do not place undo reliance on pills and powders to provide optimal nourishment. Supplements providing micronutrients (vitamins and minerals) cannot reverse the major influence of foods providing macronutrients (carbohydrate, fat, protein, fiber, water). Foods are top priority in your battle plan against diabetes.

✓ Shop the perimeter of grocery store. On the outside of your grocery store you will find fresh fruits, vegetables, bread, fish, chicken and dairy. Once you venture into the deep dark interior of the grocery store, nutritional quality of the foods goes way down and prices go way up. Organic produce is raised without pesticides and may be valuable in helping cancer patients. However, organic produce is unavailable or unaffordable for many people. Don't get terribly concerned about having to consume organic produce. Any produce that cannot be peeled (like watermelon or bananas) should be soaked for 5 minutes in a solution of one gallon lukewarm clean water with 2 tablespoons of vinegar

✓ If a food will not rot or sprout, then don't buy it, throw it out. Your body cells have similar biochemical needs to a bacteria or yeast cell. Foods that have a shelf life of a millenia are not going to nourish the body. Think about it: if bacteria is not interested in your food, then what makes you think that your body cells are interested? Foods that cannot begin (sprouting) or sustain (bacterial growth) life elsewhere, will have a similar effect in your body.

✓ Dishes should be easy to clean. Foods that are hard to digest or unhealthy will probably leave a mess on plates and pots. Dairy curd, such as fondue, is both difficult to clean and very difficult for your stomach to process. Same thing with fried, greasy or burned foods.

PATIENT PROFILE

J.T. was quite an athlete in his college days, but business luncheons and TV weekends turned his muscle into fat. It was his near-fatal heart attack that brought his doctor's attention to J.T.'s Type 2 diabetes. J.T. had 2 choices: continue the route he had been travelling, which would probably kill him within a few years, or heed my advice and begin a healthy lifestyle program. He chose the latter. Within 6 months on the diet provided in this book, J.T. lost 60 pounds, lost 12 inches around his waist, was able to resume his favorite game of tennis and was most impressed by his returned mental alertness, which brought his marriage and job into higher levels.

DR. QUILLIN'S ULTIMATE HEALTH TIPS

1. Eat God's food, not mankind's food.
2. Maintain a healthy gut environment through fiber, fluid, and probiotics.
3. Take balanced supplements in addition to, rather than instead of, good eating.
4) Minimize intake of fat, sweets, salt, and alcohol.
5) Exercise & eat to leanness--pinch an inch above the hipbone.
6) Drink lots of clean water.
7) Emphasize vegetables, whole grains, and legumes with some lean fish & poultry, fruit, and nuts.
8) Tolerance--90% nutrient dense "good" food, 10% "others".
9) Detoxify--cleanse the body and avoid poisons.
10) Live, love, laugh, learn, forgive, sing praises, seek peace.

ENDNOTES

[1]. Quillin, P., HEALING NUTRIENTS, p.43, Vintage Books, NY, 1989
[2]. Surgeon Generals Report on Nutrition and Health, p.255, US Govt. Printing Office, Washington, 1988
[3]. Patterson, BH, and Block, G., American Journal of Public Health, vol.78, p.282, Mar.1988

CHAPTER 5

NUTRITIOUS & DELICIOUS

BY NOREEN QUILLIN AND PATRICK QUILLIN

"Just a spoonful of sugar helps the medicine go down." Mary Poppins

The most important therapy for Type 2 diabetes is the proper diet. There are no drugs or vitamin supplements that can compensate for a poor diet. In this chapter you will find 2 different approaches to eating: omnivore (wide assortment of animal and plant food), and "no work" (ready to eat foods from your grocery store shelf). These recipes and menu plans are examples to get you started in the right direction. The meals outlined in this chapter are nutritious, delicious, easy to prepare, and inexpensive to buy. These foods will offer some satisfaction for your sweet tooth. We don't expect you to completely deny your desire for sweet foods. However, we are asking you to ratchet back your expectations in how sweet a food should be. Give this eating plan a 3 week trial period. It takes that long for foods to become more familiar and new patterns to replace old patterns of eating.

WHICH DIETARY PROGRAM SHOULD YOU FOLLOW?

There has been no shortage of attempts to custom tailor diets to meet the needs of specific individuals. You cannot categorize 6 billion people into only 3 or 4 dietary patterns. Dr. Weston Price observed 12 very different eating patterns that varied from high fat-high meat to smaller amounts of meat. But Dr. Price never found a completely vegan group of people. All people have consumed some small amount of animal food to provide for a more nutritious eating pattern. My recommendation?

Eat your ancestral diet

Imagine the following experiment. Dr. Rabbit, Dr. Cat and Dr. Squirrel are conducting a study of the nutrient needs of their patients, consisting of 100 subjects of 33 cats, 33 rabbits and 34 squirrels. Dr. Rabbit puts everyone on a vegetarian diet, because Dr. Rabbit is a vegan. Some of the 100 "patients" get much better, some get worse and some stay the same. Dr. Cat steps up to the plate and takes the same "mono-mania" approach of putting everyone on a carnivorous diet, just like Dr. Cat. Same results: 1/3 get better, 1/3 get worse and the rest stay the same. Dr. Squirrel has the same luck with the mixed grain and nuts diet of squirrels.

Moral of the story: there is no one perfect diet for all 6 billion people on earth. In spite of various noble efforts to categorize people based upon their blood type, their build, their nervous system type, their Ayurvedic status or whatever...you need to ask the question: "What did my ancestors eat in their native land a thousand years ago?" When I asked this question in one group of cancer patients, a person responded, "Then I guess I should be eating hog fat, like my grandpappy who was a farmer in Arkansas." I replied that, in order to give adequate credit to the adaptive forces of Nature, we need to go back further than 50 or 100 years.

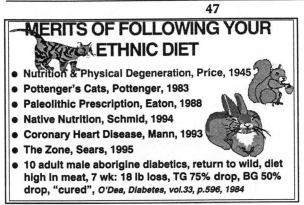

MERITS OF FOLLOWING YOUR ETHNIC DIET

- Nutrition & Physical Degeneration, Price, 1945
- Pottenger's Cats, Pottenger, 1983
- Paleolithic Prescription, Eaton, 1988
- Native Nutrition, Schmid, 1994
- Coronary Heart Disease, Mann, 1993
- The Zone, Sears, 1995
- 10 adult male aborigine diabetics, return to wild, diet high in meat, 7 wk: 18 lb loss, TG 75% drop, BG 50% drop, "cured", *O'Dea, Diabetes, vol.33, p.596, 1984*

Basically, if you are very weak and have no one to cook for you, then use the ready to eat cooking concept, until you can regain enough strength to begin cooking. If your ancestors came from a warm and sunny climate, then they probably ate more plant food, which is available year round in the warmer climates, and less animal food. If your ancestors came from a colder climate, then you probably need more lean and clean animal food along with healthy amounts of unprocessed plant food. How many people from Scandinavia and Great Britain were vegetarians 1000 years ago?

TO LOSE WEIGHT

♥ Never say "diet". This program must be a lifetime effort, with occasional "holidays" to eat outside of these boundaries.

♥ Eat 6 smaller meals a day.

♥ Have warm fluids, like tea or soup, about 20 minutes before mealtime.

♥ Use a smaller plate. It gives the illusion that you are eating more. Drink plenty of purified water. It's good for both weight loss, constipation and wrinkles.

♥ Exercise within your ability. Make sure you enjoy it.

♥ Eat more high-fiber foods, such as fruits, vegetables, beans and whole-grain cereals.

♥ Plan ahead for your meals and snacks instead of waiting until you are hungry and then eating convenient junk food.

EATING OUT

♥ Salad bars can be a great place to nourish yourself. Iceberg lettuce is the most common salad bar offering, but is "junk food" relative to most other vegetables. A good rule of thumb: the deeper the color of the vegetable, the more nourishing it is. Dark greens are better than pale greens, dark orange squash is better than pale squash, and so on.

♥ Many restaurants offer low-calorie or light meals with gourmet versions.

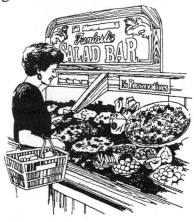

♥ Instead of accepting that "fried" meal from a restaurant menu, most places will steam or broil your food.

♥ Airlines can be very accommodating in having a special meal ready for you. Give them at least 1 week advance notice.

♥ Ask for the salad dressing to be served on the side.

♥ Have the rich sauces or gravies left out.

♥ Avoid sauteed and deep-fried food.

JUICING VERSUS PUREEING. Juicing has its advantages, because one glass of carrot juice is equal to about a pound of carrots, which few of us could eat. Unfortunately, much of the valuable nutrients in the vegetables get tossed out with the pulp that is discarded. That is why I recommend that you puree rather than juice the vegetable or fruit. There are 10 times more body-strengthening agents in pureed whole vegetables than in juice extracted from vegetable pulp.

BEVERAGES TO HIGHLIGHT

-Purified water
-Cafix
-Roma
-Herb tea
-Vitamin C powder & honey in hot water
-Ginger tea
-Hot natural apple juice with vitamin C
-Fresh orange juice
-Postum
-Chickory
-Japanese Green tea
-Roasted rice or barley tea
-Vinegar, honey & water

SUGAR

The more you eliminate white table sugar and other high risk sweeteners (see chapter on "sweeteners") from your diet, the healthier you will be.

Substitutes for 1 Cup White Sugar		Reduce Liquids by
Honey	1/2 cup	1/8 to 1/4 cup
Fructose	1/3 to 1/2 cup	
Molasses	1/2 cup	1/4 cup
Mashed ripe banana	1 cup	
Sucanat	3/4 cup	
Maple Sugar	1/2 cup	
	1/4 cup	
Apple or other fruit juice	1 cup	1/4 cup
Splenda (sucralose)	1 cup	1 cup

Stevia (herbal concentrate) follow label directions for dilution in water. It is 25 times sweeter than sugar

Splenda has zero calories; you can bake with it; use where you would sugar. You can only order it through the internet, http://www.sucralose.com It is a product by Johnson & Johnson. You must be over 18 years old with diabetes or a family member to order this product at this time.

-Vanilla, cinnamon, and cardamon can be used to replace sugar toppings and in dessert sauces. Cinnamon is a valuable condiment and herb to help reduce blood sugar levels.

Desserts are given at the end of each dinner. This doesn't mean we want you to always have a dessert! Try and keep sweets to a minimum. Try using a piece of fruit (i.e. cherries, blueberries, grapefruit) and a few almonds for the end of the meal. Make a game out of lowering the sugar in your diet. Have a weekly "prize" or non edible treat for a reward.

FATS

GOOD FATS
Kitchen: olive oil, canola, lecithin, vegetable spray oils (i.e. Pam), MCT oil, and better butter (1/2 butter & 1/2 canola or olive oil whipped together).
Therapeutic: fish, flax, borage, evening primrose, grape seed, hemp, black current, pumpkin

BAD FATS
oxidized (over used), hydrogenated, saturated, too much corn or soy oil

IDEAS TO REPLACE FAT
Marinate without fat by using lemon, orange, tomato, yogurt & juice with herbs, sauces, tomato with onions and garlic, vegetable stock
Saute in water, stock, vegetable bouillon, juice, liquid instead of fat
Steam cook or microwave vegetables
Steam bake corn tortillas in oven instead of frying

-Crackers often contain large amounts of hydrogenated fats
-Use 2 teaspoons of canola or olive oil in place of 1 tablespoon shortening
-Butter is better than margarine
-Use raised broiler pan in oven so the excess fat will drop away
-Avoid processed meats, like bologna and salami
Dairy:
-Low fat or non fat plain yogurt vs. sour cream; no fat cream cheese; substitute with lowfat
-Salad dressings usually use fat as main ingredients
-Delicious lowfat garlic bread: coat bread with butter flavor Pam and sprinkle with garlic powder. Bake 5-10 minutes at 350 degrees.
-Foods that taste fried but aren't: Dip chicken in whipped egg. Then dip in sack with whole wheat cracker crumbs, oat flour, corn meal, and spices. Spray with Pam. Bake 400 degrees for 1 hour, turning every 20 minutes, spraying with Pam.

Some More Kitchen Tips

⇒ Better Butter. Make Better Butter by whipping together: 1/2 cup olive oil and 1/2 cup butter. Refrigerate.
⇒ Prepare food ahead. You might have more energy on certain days than others.
⇒ A pressure cooker is a must. Cook in bulk. Good items to have on hand are: beans, rice, refried beans, etc.
⇒ Crock pots are very handy to have in the kitchen. You just place the ingredients into to pot in the morning and by evening, the meal is ready.
⇒ Using liquid lecithin. Measure it by your eye. It's hard to get off a measuring spoon. If you do want to measure with a utensil, put a bit of oil on the utensil first. You can use liquid lecithin for a thickening agent if you are substituting. Too much will make dough gummy. Pam is basically aerosol lecithin. That's good.

⇒ Look for lecithin in spray vegetable oil. There are some that have olive oil also.

⇒ Measuring honey. Measure the oil first. The honey will just slide out of the measuring cup.

⇒ The garlic recipe is one to have as often as possible. You might find that if you have it with dinner, you are energized and might not be able to fall asleep easily. Switch the time to lunch.

⇒ To remove pesticide residue from fresh produce: Soak produce that cannot be peeled in a gallon of tepid water and 1-2 Tbs. cheap vinegar. Leave for about 5 minutes, then rinse off.

⇒ Leave peeled baby carrots in purified water in the refrigerator. This will make them sweeter.

⇒ Sweeten desserts by adding extra cinnamon and vanilla.

⇒ Grow alfalfa sprouts. It's fun to watch them grow and you know they are organic. It only takes about a week.

⇒ Buy baking powder without alum in it.

⇒ You can add flax meal to salads and vegetables. Just sprinkle a bit on the top for a nice change of flavor.

⇒ Use leftovers for breakfast meals.

⇒ Grow a pot of parsley in the kitchen. It's great to have on hand when you serve onions or garlic.

⇒ You can use unsweetened applesauce to replace 1/2 amount of oil in dessert recipes and add 1/4 to 1/2 tsp. lecithin.

⇒ Become a Label Reader! Check and see if that whole wheat bread lists "enriched flour" as first ingredient. Beware of "fat free". See if sugar was added. Limit saturated fat and sugar. Sugar can be listed as: maltose, dextrose, fructose, sucrose, corn syrup, date sugar, etc.

Growing Your Sprouts

Sprouts can be a great way of having organic produce growing in your kitchen year round without any dirt. You will need a glass jar (quart size or larger), a soft plastic screen for the top, and a rubber band to hold the screen in place. There are also commercial sprouting kits available in most health food stores. Place about one heaping tablespoon of seeds in your glass container with the screen doubled on the top. The seeds will expand about tenfold as they sprout, so allow enough room for their expansion. Fill the container half full of purified water and let stand overnight. Next morning drain and rinse the seeds. Let stand inverted over the sink for proper drainage. Rinse and drain twice each day for the next 6-7 days. Keep the jar in a dimly lit area.

Larger seeds, like peas, beans, and lentils take a shorter time to grow and should not be allowed to grow more than a half inch long, since they will develop a bitter flavor. Mung bean sprouts can get up to two inches in length without bitter flavor. Wheat, barley, oats, and other grass plants make terrific sprouts. Smaller seeds, like alfalfa, can grow to an inch in length without any bitter flavor. For some extra vitamin A, let the alfalfa sprouts sit in a sunny window for the last day before eating. The green color indicates the welcome addition of chlorophyll, folacin and beta-carotene.

Fast Breakfast Ideas

-hard boiled eggs
-low sugar protein bar
-whole grain cereals, without the sugar
added,with juice or milk
-oatmeal bagel with no fat cream cheese or natural peanut
butter
-instant oatmeal with powder protein or rice bran added
-non-fat, low-fat yogurt, without the fruit & with active
probiotic

RECIPES

There are two different recipe formats. Monday is a day of no work cooking. You can become a good label reader and find companies making healthy fast foods that can be used sparingly. The rest are for Omnivores (meat,poultry and fish). These will give you an idea of meal preparation using minimal sweetners.

The salad dressing used is one you can made that is healthy for your body.

ROYAL SALAD DRESSING

1/4 cup each of apple cider vinegar, flax oil, olive oil, & water
1 package dry Italian Salad Dressing Mix (i.e. Good Seasons)
1-2 tsp. liquid lecithin

Add all ingredients together in a jar with a lid. Shake vigorously. Keep refrigerated

---

MONDAY (ready to eat foods, no work)

Breakfast

Ready to eat healthy cereal (i.e. Shredded Wheat, Grapenuts, Grapenut flakes, Cheerios).
Serve with skim milk or apple juice.
Country Farms stone ground whole wheat toast with:
Simply fruit spread jam or Smuckers Natural Style reduced fat peanut butter.
Louis Rich Turkey-ham slices
Fresh cherry tomatoes.

Lunch

Fantastic Foods Hummus Mix
International Mr. Pita 100% whole wheat pita bread
Janet Lee California pitted ripe olives

Sliced fresh red onion or spring onion
Ready to eat carrots, soaked in purified water

Dinner
Hormell's Turkey Chili
Uncle Ben's Brown & Wild Rice
Fresh vegetable platter served with *Royal Salad Dressing

TUESDAY (omnivore eating days)
Breakfast:
This can be made the night before.

Rice Milk
1/4 cup brown rice
1 1/4 quarts of purified water
1/8 tsp. sea salt
1 1/2 Tbs. honey
1/2 Tbs. canola oil
 Bring rice and water to a boil; then simmer for 45
minutes. Strain the rice, saving the liquid, and add back 1/4
cup of the liquid. Add the salt, honey and oil. Whip in a
blender on high. Add back to fluid. Chill. Shake before using.

**Variation: For a glass of "unchocolate milk", mix 8 ounces
of rice milk with 2 Tbs. of carob powder (chocolate flavor) and
1/2 Tbs. of Roma (coffee substitute). Use
electric blender for 10 seconds.
Serve chilled.

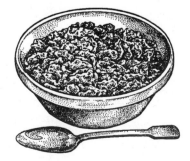

Granola
4 cups old-fashioned oats,
uncooked
1/4 cup unprocessed rice bran
1/4 cup wheat germ
1/2 cup oat bran

1/4 cup canola oil
2 Tbs. honey
1/2 to 1 cup sunflower seeds
1/3 cup raisins
2 tsp. vanilla

Heat oven to 300 degrees. Mix together the first 6 ingredients. Spread into a large, shallow pan. Bake for 45 minutes, stirring every 15 minutes. Add the sunflower seeds during the last 10 minutes of baking. Add the raisins and vanilla at the end of the baking time. Let cool.

Lunch

Bacon, Tomato, Spinach Sandwich

Turkey bacon, cooked
tomato slices
spinach leaves, cleaned
100% whole wheat sourdough bread, toasted

On toast, layer the bacon, tomato, and spinach leaves. Can spread toast with *Royal Salad Dressing or mayonnaise.

Own Mayonnaise

1 block soft tofu
3 Tbs. flax oil
3 Tbs. apple cider vinegar
salt to taste
your favorite seasoning (opt.)

Place the ingredients in a blender and puree until smooth.

Cabbage Pecan Salad

1 1/2 cups finely shredded green cabbage
1/4 cup red seedless grapes, halved (opt.)
1/4 cup red apple, diced
1/4 cup pineapple, diced (opt.)
1 Tbs. chopped pecans

Place the cabbage in a serving bowl. Add the rest of the ingredients. Toss. Serve with *Royal Salad Dressing.

Dinner

Easy Chicken & Sweet Potato Dinner

2-4 chicken breasts, washed
Onion powder
Spike seasoning or:
Lowery's seasoning without MSG
2-4 medium sweet potatoes or yams

Place sweet potatoes that have been pierced with a knife in a foil-lined pan. In a 375 degrees preheated oven, cook the sweet potatoes for fifteen to minutes. Then add the chicken that has been placed in a foil lined baking dish and sprinkled with the seasonings. Bake for 45 to 50 minutes more. If the sweet potatoes are large, you can microwave them for 4 or 5 minutes before placing in oven.

Delicious Garlic

1 bulb/head of garlic
Spike, or your favorite seasonings
1 tsp. olive oil
soy sauce

Cut the garlic head through the center. Break up the pieces. Place in a glass cup and sprinkle with olive oil, teriyaki sauce and seasonings. Microwave for 1 minute.

Carrots with Bean Sprouts

2 large carrots, shredded
2 cups alfalfa sprouts
1 cup bean sprouts
1/2 cup walnuts or pecans
1/4 cup sliced almonds
2 Tbs. white-wine vinegar

2 tsp. Dijon-style mustard (opt.)
1 Tbs. sesame oil
1 Tbs. olive oil
salt and pepper
2 tsp. chopped fresh coriander, parsley, or dill
  Mix the carrots, sprouts, and nuts together and place in a serving dish. Blend the rest of ingredients together. Pour over the salad. Or you can use *Royal Salad Dressing.

   Cherries Jubilee
1 qt. apple juice or cherry juice
1/3 cup agar flakes (find it in health food stores)
1 lb. cherries, halved and pitted
1 tsp. Vanilla
dash of cinnamon (opt.)
pinch of sugar
  Pour apple juice into a pot and add agar. Stir and bring to a boil over medium heat. Simmer 15 to 20 minutes until agar is dissolved. Add vanilla and cherries. Simmer 5 minutes. Remove from heat. Pour into bowls. Cool and refrigerate.

WEDNESDAY

Breakfast
  Blended drink of pureed carrots in orange juice with added powdered protein and 1/2 frozen peeled banana
  Grapenuts or favorite non-sweetened cereal with non-fat milk or unsweetened apple juice
  1/4 to 1/2 cup cherries, or 1/2 grapefruit

Lunch
  Tuna Cakes
6 ounces water-packed tuna, drained
6 whole grain crackers, finely crushed
1/4 cup oats
1/4 cup minced red bell pepper

2 Tbs. fresh, minced parsley
2 Tbs. minced onions
1 egg
2 tsp. yogurt or water
1 1/2 tsp. lemon juice
1 tsp. Worcestershire
1/8 tsp. ground red pepper or 1/4 tsp. chili powder
1-2 tsp. minced fresh basil
1/2 tsp. marjoram
1 clove garlic, minced
No stick cooking spray

    Spray a frying pan with the oil. In large bowl, gently mix all ingredients. Using scant 1/4 cup mixture for each, make 6 cakes. Shape mixture into circle, pressing flat. (If they are too dry to hold a shape, add a bit more water.) Place in frying pan and fry on both sides until golden brown. Serve with a whole wheat roll.
Serves two.

Spice Beets
2 cups cooked beets, grated
1/4 cup water
1/3 cup vinegar
1/2 to 1 Tbs. fructose
1/2 tsp. cinnamon
1/4 tsp. cloves
1/4 tsp. salt

    Mix all ingredients together and simmer 7-10 minutes.

Dinner
Spicy Mexican Beans
2 cups pinto beans
1 large onion, diced
4 cloves garlic, minced
2-3 dry red peppers, minced (can cut with scissors)

1 Tbs. chili powder
1 tsp. cumin powder
1/4 cup olive oil or canola oil
2 tsp. sea salt
purified water

Sort and wash beans in a colander. Place beans in a pressure cooker and add enough water to cover the beans and then 4 cups more. Bring to a boil and boil for 2 minutes. Cover and leave for 1 hour. Drain and rinse beans. Place beans back into the pressure cooker and add water to just cover the beans. Add the rest of ingredients and close lid. Heat on high until the weight starts rocking. Turn down the heat but keep the weight moving for 25 minutes. Turn off heat. Let the pressure cooker sit until the indicator shows that all pressure has been released. Remove lid and mash the beans with an egg beater until about 1/2 of the beans are mashed.

If you don't want to use a pressure cooker, follow the steps except when placing the beans with the rest of the ingredients, place the beans and ingredients in a large pot and let boil for about 90-120 minutes or until beans are tender. More water will be needed.

To give you a few ideas, these beans can be used to make: burritos, tacos, a bean sandwich with a slice of onion on top,or a hot dip with baked corn chips.

Spanish Rice
Cooked brown rice
Salsa to desired amount
Spring onions sliced
chopped fresh parsley

Mix all ingredients together and heat in the microwave.

Whole wheat tortillas

Fruit & Sprout Salad

1 ripe pear or banana
3 to 4 drops Stevia
3 apples, grated
2-3 Tbs. lemon juice
1 cup germinated sunflower seeds
1 cup wheat sprouts or alfalfa sprouts
1/2 cup wheat germ
Chopped almonds

In a large bowl, mash the pear or banana with Stevia. Add the next 2 ingredients and mix well. Fold in next 3 ingredients. Serve in individual bowls and top with chopped almond. (Makes 4 generous servings.)

THURSDAY

Breakfast

Slice banana bread (low in sugar)
Turkey bacon cooked
Tomato slices

Lunch

Pita Bread Sandwich

Fill a pita pocket with some of the following and sprinkle with *Royal Salad Dressing if appropriate:
tomato slices
grated carrot
natural peanut or almond butter
raisins
mashed banana
low-fat cheese
sprouts
avocado slices
spinach leaves
sliced mushrooms

Deviled Eggs

4 hard-boiled eggs, peeled and cut in half lengthwise
1-2 tsp. mayonnaise or ranch salad dressing
1/2 tsp. prepared mustard
1 tsp. pickle relish
dash of onion powder
salt and pepper to taste

Remove yolks from eggs and mash. Set aside egg white halves. Mix yolks with remaining ingredients. Spoon mixture into egg whites. Garnish tops with a dash of paprika.

Dinner

Sesame Chicken

4 split chicken breasts, skinned and boned
1/2 Tbs. lemon pepper
1 tsp. basil
1/2 tsp. garlic, chopped
2 eggs lightly beaten
1/4 cup oat flour or barley flour
1/8 cup sesame seeds

Wash chicken and remove all visible fat. Place chicken in a zip lock bag with lemon pepper, basil and garlic and eggs and coat the chicken. Mix oat flour and sesame seeds together. Dip each piece of marinated chicken in the flour mixture and place meat side up in a baking dish that has been sprayed with vegetable oil (i.e. Pam) or you can use oven paper. Spray the chicken with the vegetable oil. Bake at 350 degrees for 45-50 minutes spraying spraying the chicken 25 minutes into the cooking time.

Delicious Garlic

1 bulb/head of garlic
Spike, or your favorite seasonings
1 tsp. olive oil
soy sauce or low sugar teriyaki sauce

Cut the garlic head through the center. Break up the pieces. Place in a glass cup and sprinkle with olive oil, soy or teriyaki sauce and seasonings. Microwave for 1 minute.

Stir-Fried Spinach with Ginger
1 lb. fresh spinach
1 small onion
1 Tbs. olive oil
1 clove garlic, minced fine
1/2 Tbs. ginger, finely minced
1 Tbs. soy sauce
1 tsp. honey

Wash and trim spinach and cut leaves into wide strips. Chop onion. Heat oil and add onion, garlic, and ginger. Stir-fry on high heat for 1 minute. Add spinach and stir for just a few minutes. Add soy sauce and honey; turn down heat and cook about 1-2 minutes longer.

Broiled Apple Rings
4 small apples
1 packet Splenda or Steviia
1/2 tsp. Cinnamon

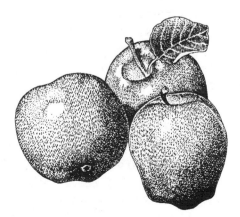

Wash apples and slice into 1/2 inch rounds. Core each slice. In a cup combine the sugar substitute and cinnamon. Place rings on a greased cookie sheet and broil for 8 minutes or until light brown. With a spatula, gently turn each ring. Sprinkle with the cinnamon mixture and broil for one more minute. Serve hot or cold.

FRIDAY

Breakfast

Oat Raisin Scones

1 cup oats
1 cup whole wheat flour
1 Tbs. fructose
1 1/2 tsp. baking powder
1/4 tsp. soda
1/8 tsp. salt (opt.)
1/4 cup raisins
1/4 cup canola oil
1/2 cup unsweetened applesauce
1/4 to 1/2 tsp. liquid lecithin
1 Tbs lemon juice
1/4 tsp. cinnamon (opt.)
1 egg

Blend together the dry ingredients. Add the raisins.
Combine the rest of the ingredients. Mix.   Turn dough out
onto a lightly floured surface. Flour your hands. Dough might
be a bit sticky. Don't add too much flour or it will toughen the
scones. You can use a spatula to help in the kneading.   Knead
until about 8-10 turns. Divide dough into two equal parts. Pat
each part into a circle 1/2 inch thick. Cut into quarters.
Transfer onto a baking sheet sprayed with vegetable oil or lined
with oven paper. Bake until golden, about 20-25 minutes in
400 degree preheated oven. The scones can make a great
dessert by serving warm and sprinkling a bit of fructose with
cinnamon on the top.

1 egg - poached or boiled
1 glass orange juice

Lunch

Fast Pizzas

1 whole wheat pita bread

fresh tomato slices
thinly sliced onion rings
green pepper, diced
sliced black olives (opt.)
sliced mushrooms (opt.)
leftover protein (i.e. dice turkey, sausage, bacon, etc.)
oregano
light olive oil, sprinkled over vegetables
grated low fat cheese

You can use oven paper on a cookie sheet. Top bread with items listed. Baked in preheated 375 degree oven for about 8 to 10 minutes or until cheese is bubbly.

Spinach and Peeled Grapefruit Salad
spinach leaves
fresh peeled or canned grapefruit
nuts, chopped

Place cleaned spinach in individual serving bowls. Place grapefruit sections with some of the juice on the top of the spinach. Can sprinkle a bit of coconut, chopped nuts or seeds on the top.

Dinner
Pressure Cooked Beef
3-4 pounds of lean roast (i.e. London Broiler)
1/3 pkg. of dry onion soup mix
1 cup water, wine, or vegetable stock
fresh onion slices

Place the beef on the rack in the pressure cooker. Add the soup mix and fluid. Place onion slices on top. Bring the pressure cooker to a rock. Rock for 25 minutes. Turn off the heat. Let the steam valve go down on it's own.

Carrot and Cabbage Salad
2 cups grated carrots

2 cups grated cabbage
1 spring onion chopped (opt.)
　　Mix together and cover with *Royal Salad Dressing.

Basil Pesto

1 cup fresh basil leaves
1 1/2 cup spinach leaves
2 garlic cloves
1 Tbs. pine nuts or walnuts
2 Tbs. Parmesan cheese
1/2 Tbs. olive oil
2 Tbs. water
　　Add all ingredients together in a blender. Process until a smooth paste. Use spatula and off/on motions to help processing. If you don't want to add the cheese, cut the water to 1 Tbs. Serve on stoneground whole wheat rolls or crackers.

Oatmeal Raisin Cookies

3 cups uncooked oatmeal
1 cup whole wheat flour
1 tsp. cinnamon
1/2 tsp. nutmeg
1/2 tsp. baking soda
1/2 cup unsweetened applesauce
1/2 cup canola
1/4 to 1/2 tsp. liquid lecithin (opt.)
2 tsp. vanilla
1 egg
1/2 cup chopped nuts (opt.)
1 to 2 Tbs. raisins
　　Heat oven to 375 degrees. Lightly spray cookie sheet with no stick cooking spray or use oven paper. Combine dry ingredients, mixing well. Mix the rest of the ingredients stirring until well mixed. Place rounded spoonfuls of mixture on the cookie sheet. Bake approximately 10 to 12 minutes until

golden brown. If you want a sweeter taste, you could add a couple packets of Splenda or Stevia to the mixture.

SATURDAY

Breakfast
100% whole wheat bagel with no-fat cream cheese
egg fried with pan sprayed in Pam
baby carrots soaked in purified water
1/2 grapefruit

Lunch
Ground Beef Stuffed Potatoes
2 hot baked sweet potatoes (can be cooked in the microwave)
1/4 cup hot skim milk or rice milk
1 green onion, minced
1 egg
2 tsp. butter or canola oil
1/4 tsp. salt
1/2 tsp. black pepper
1/2 cup diced tomato
cooked ground beef
2 tsp. Parmesan cheese, grated (opt.)

Cut a thin slice off the top of each baked potato, scoop out potato and combine with hot milk, green onion, beaten egg and butter. Whip well. Add salt, pepper and gently stir in tomato and beef. Fill potato skins with this mixture by mounding it high. Sprinkle with Parmesan cheese. Place on baking sheet and cook at 400 degrees for 10-15 minutes.

Colorful Salad
Spinach leaves
alfalfa sprouts
carrots, grated
pickled beets, grated

edible flower (i.e. pansy) opt.

On a bed of spinach leaves, place some sprouts, carrots and pickled beets. Sprinkle with *Royal Salad Dressing and place a flower on the top.

Dinner
Spicy Turkey Loaf
1 cup onion (large) diced
1/2 cup green pepper, diced
2 cloves garlic, minced
1/2 tsp. black pepper
1 piece whole wheat bread, cubed
1 egg
1 tsp. liquid lecithin
1 tsp. Worcestershire sauce
1/4 tsp. Tabasco
1 tsp. Spike, or dry poultry seasoning
1 tsp. dry oregano
1 Tbs. chopped parsley
12 ounces tomato sauce
1 pound raw ground turkey

Preheat oven to 425 degrees. Mix all ingredients reserving 1/2 cup tomato sauce. Spray a 4x8 loaf pan with vegetable coating spray and place mixture in pan. Pat down until firm and top with remaining sauce. Bake at 425 degrees for 1 hour until lightly browned around edges.

Raw Cauliflower Salad
1 cup raw cauliflower, grated
1 cup raw tender garden peas
1/2 cup avocado, diced
green pepper
couple of black olives (opt.)

Toss with *Royal Salad Dressing. Serve on spinach leaves. Garnish with green pepper strips and olives for color contrast.

Microwave garlic

1 bulb of garlic
1 tsp. Teriyaki sauce (opt.)
olive oil
Spike

Cut garlic bulb in half through the equator. Break up bulb into pieces and place in a glass cup. Drizzle olive oil and teriyaki on top and sprinkle with spike. Place a piece of plastic wrap over the top of the cup and microwave for 1 minute. The skins of the garlic just fall off.

Apple Bread Pudding

3 slices whole wheat bread, cubed
1 1/2 Tbs. chopped walnuts or pecans (opt.)
3 small apples, peeled and chopped
1/4 cup unsweetened apple juice
3 eggs
3/4 cup non fat plain yogurt or unsweetened applesauce
1/4 to1/2 tsp. lecithin
1/4 tsp. ground cinnamon
1 tsp. vanilla

Preheat oven to 350 degrees. Sprinkle bread cubes and walnuts into a square pan coated with non-stick cooking spray. Sprinkle with chopped apples; set aside. Beat together apple juice, eggs, yogurt, lecithin, cinnamon and vanilla until smooth; pour over bread and fruit in pan. Bake for 30 minutes. Press apples down into custard with spatula and bake an additional 20 minutes until custard is set. Serve warm or cold.

SUNDAY

Brunch

Scrambled Eggs with Rice

4 eggs
1 cup cooked brown rice or wild rice, (not hot)
2 Tbs. skim milk or water
1 tsp. Worcestershire
1 Tbs. Parmesan cheese (opt.)
1/4 tsp. oregano
1 tsp. parsley
2 tsp. salsa

Combine all ingredients in a bowl. Stir ingredients until well blended. Lightly coat a nonstick skillet with better butter (recipe in "Kitchen Tips") and place over medium heat. Pour in egg mixture. Scramble the eggs until they are cooked. The mixture will still be moist. Serve with extra salsa.

Serve with:
Turkey bacon, cooked
Whole wheat tortillas
Tomato slices

Dinner

Easy Salmon Dinner

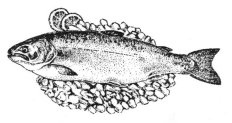

1-2 pound salmon filet or steak
Low sugar Teriyaki sauce

Turn on broiler. Place salmon on broiler pan sprayed with vegetable oil where you will be placing the salmon. Broil on one side for about 8 minutes. Flip. Spread the teriyaki sauce on the top of salmon. Bake another 8 minutes or until done. You might have to move the fish to a lower shelf so the top doesn't burn. If you are broiling halibut or a less oily fish, you can put foil on the broiling pan to save on clean up time.

If you don't have access to fresh fish:

Salmon Cakes

1 can (14.75 oz) salmon
1 cup dry oatmeal cereal
2 eggs
1/2 Tbs. lemon juice
2 tsp. minced parsley
1 tsp. onion powder

      Drain salmon. Skim off skin and bones. Mix all ingredients. Make into patties. Fry in 2 tsp. olive oil or canola oil. When brown, flip and brown other side.

Tomato & Red Onion Salad

Sliced tomatoes
Thinly sliced red onion, seperate rings

      Alternate sliced tomatoes and onions. Can top with:
-grated parmesan cheese
-basil
-fresh herbs
-sunflower seeds
-*Royal Salad Dressing

Brown Rice Delight

2 cups cooked instant brown rice or cooked brown rice
1 apple, diced
1-2 Tbs. walnuts or pecans, chopped
1-2 Tbs. raisins
2 Tbs celery leaves,chopped
1 tsp. poultry seasoning

      Mix all ingredients together. Add a few teaspoons of water if too dry. Microwave for 1 minute.

Chewy Carrot Brownies

3/4 cup barley flour or whole wheat flour
1 tsp. baking powder

1 cup rolled oats
1/4 cup raisins
1 cup shredded carrots
1/4 cup fructose
1/3 cup canola oil
1/2 tsp. liquid lecithin
1/4 cup unsweetened applesauce
1 tsp. maple extract (opt.)

Preheat oven to 375 degrees. In bowl mix dry ingredients together. In separate bowl, stir together liquid ingredients, carrots and raisins. Stir into dry ingredients until well moistened. Add a little bit of applesauce if batter is too stiff. Place in a greased 8x8 square pan. Bake for about 25 minutes until slightly browned. Can also make the dough into cookies and bake for 10-12 minutes or until golden brown on top. May add nuts or sunflower seeds when adding the raisins.

PATIENT PROFILE

M.V. had been an award winning chef in a major city restaurant when the overeating pushed her into Type 2 diabetes. She already had the beginnings of blurred vision and tingling in the feet when she passed out one night at work. M.V. loved to cook and eat and was distressed when I suggested a new way of eating. However, once she tried some of these recipes, she found an enjoyment that was not found in her heavy sauces. "Clean and unadulterated" food became her motto. Demand for her services at other restaurants brought her a raise and fame with her "low fat, low sugar, high taste" cuisine. Her blood glucose and body weight are both within reason and she no longer has problems with poor circulation in her feet or eyes.

CHAPTER 6

SUPER FOODS
FOR DIABETES IMPROVEMENT

"The excessive use of sugar as a food is usually considered one of the causes of diabetes." Encylopaedia Britannica, 1911

While there are no magic bullets to cure diabetes, there are several "superfoods" that can dramatically improve the quantity and quality of life for the diabetic. These foods are a rich and complex array of phytochemicals, special fatty acids, vitamins, minerals, and other unknown "sub-nutrients" that improve blood glucose regulation, enhance insulin activity, and slow down the complications of diabetes.

FISH

Deep clean coldwater fish is on just about every nutritionists list for a "superfood". Fish is not only rich in protein, vitamin B-6, B-12, and trace minerals from the sea; but 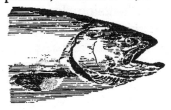 fish also contains the missing fat in the American diet: omega 3. In one study, people who consumed less than an ounce of fish daily, or 7 ounces weekly, had a significant reduction in their incidence of glucose intolerance along with a general 50% reduction in mortality.[1] If you absolutely cannot stand the taste of fresh

fish, then try taking capsule supplements of fish, such as
SeaCure (800-555-8868).

Small amounts of clean cold water fish, such as salmon,
halibut, sole, cod, tuna, trout, sardines, and others can
dramatically protect the diabetic from the complications of the
disease.[2] Fish oil provides a crucial nutrient to the delicate cell
membranes, which then are better able to receive insulin and
allow for glucose to pass into the cell. Our ancestors used to
eat a diet of about 20% fat with a ratio of 1 to 1 of omega 3 to
omega 6 oils and no hydrogenated (trans) fats. Our current
American diet provides about 40% of calories from fat with a 1
to 30 ratio of omega 3 to omega 6 fats and frightening levels of
trans fats to confuse the cell membrane insulin receptors.
Avoid hydrogenated fats like Crisco and margarine. Consume
fresh fish and take fish oil or flax oil supplements. See the
"nutritious & delicious" chapter for a blue ribbon "Blue Ribbon
diabetes buster" salad dressing that is so powerful at controlling
blood glucose levels you should need a prescription to get it--
but you don't.

VINEGAR

Real vinegar has not been filtered or pasteurized, and is
rich in organic acids, mother of vinegar "friendly" bacteria,
pectin (soluble fiber), and acetic acid all of which help to slow
down the emptying of the stomach. This simple "detour" for
the digestion of food creates a slowdown in dumping glucose
into the bloodstream. A meal with 2 tablespoons of vinegar
can slow gastric emptying rate by 30% and drop blood glucose
peaks by 30%.[3] Check out the "nutritious & delicious" chapter
for a fabulous "Blue Ribbon diabetes buster" recipe for salad
dressing with flax oil and vinegar that not only tastes great but
can dramatically improve overall health by lowering rises in
blood glucose. Red wine vinegar works best at this
hypoglycemic role.

COLORFUL VEGETABLES

Free radicals, or prooxidants, have been labeled the "age inducers" of the human body. Free radicals steal electrons from tissue, like your heart, blood vessels, brain, cell membrane and DNA; leading you toward premature aging and diseases. This destructive process is accelerated in diabetics. Antioxidants block the destruction caused by free radicals and 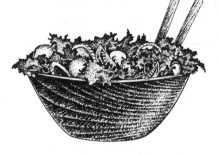 the richest sources of mixed antioxidants are in colorful fruits and vegetables. The reasons for this cornucopia of antioxidants is that plants must stay out in the damaging free radical bombardment of the sun and need some protection. The "sun protective tanning agents" are colorful pigments in plants. These pigments that protect the plant from the damaging effects of the sun can become a bulletproof vest for you in your quest to retard the free radical production found in diabetics.

There are over 20,000 known bioflavonoids (such as quercetin from onions) and over 800 different carotenoids (such as beta carotene from carrots). Together, these bioflavonoids and carotenoids form a tight network of antioxidants to corral the damaging effects of free radicals. Much of the complications from diabetes come from the stepped up free radical production as a consequence of too much glucose in the bloodstream.

Therefore, spinach and collards are more nutrient dense in these pigment antioxidants than iceberg lettuce. The darker the red of the tomato, the richer the antioxidant content. Red grapes are better than white grapes. Raspberries and boysenberries even have their own pigment antioxidant, ellagic acid, that has piqued the interest of the National Institutes of Health for its ability to control unwanted growth in the body.

Mix up a huge salad bowl of colorful vegetables and keep it covered in the refrigerator. Scoop up a bowl of these colorful veggies at most of your meals.

BREWER'S YEAST

In order for glucose to get inside the human cell, there must be two "doormen" available: Glucose Tolerance Factor, a molecule that contains niacin and chromium, along with the more famous doorman, insulin. In many Type 2 diabetics, lacking the GTF doorman brings on elevated blood glucose and a casade of problems. The richest food source of GTF is brewer's yeast. Mix a tablespoon of this grainy, nutty tasting powder into a blended shake of orange juice, powdered protein, flax oil, and lecithin. In 10-20% of Type 2 diabetics, this food alone can substantially reduce glucose levels for Type 2 diabetics.

FLAX

With respect to fats, the statement "You are what you eat" is exactly true. The fats in your body, brain, insulation for nerve cells, cell membranes, and prostaglandins all comes from your diet. If your diet is high in hard fats, like saturated fats from margarine and beef, then the fats in your cell membranes are more rigid. If your diet is rich in highly unsaturated fats from fish and flax oil, then your cell membranes become more flexible and are better able to perform their duties.

Our ancestors ate a diet that was approximately 1 to 1 ratio of to omega 6 fats (soy, corn, safflower) to omega 3 fats (fish and flax). We now eat a diet that contains a ratio of 30 to 1 omega 6 fats to omega 3 fats.[4] This mind boggling imbalance has brought a host of diseases, including cancer, heart disease, infections, arthritis, and diabetes.

Diabetes oftentimes originates when the cell membrane does not recognize the insulin outside, though there may be plenty of insulin. Lack of omega 3 fats from fish and flax can be the cause of this improper construction of the cell membrane insulin receptor. While the intake of fish has been closely related to preventing and slowing diabetes, the intake of fish oil is a bit more complex. Possibly because of the varying levels of saturated fats in fish oil capsules or due to the presence of rusted fats (lipid peroxides), fish oil capsules have had mixed results as supplements in diabetics. In a few studies with diabetics, fish oil supplements that were highly processed (removed cholesterol & vitamins) deteriorated blood fats, glucose, and insulin sensitivity, while in other studies fish oil capsules (pure cod liver oil) improved these same parameters.

However, flax oil, contains alpha linolenic acid which can be converted into fish oil (eicosapentaenoic acid) in the body. Flax oil is lower in lipid peroxides, cheaper, and tastes much better than fish oil. See the recipe chapter for a fabulous salad dressing with flax oil.

CINNAMON

When researchers at the United States Department of Agriculture (USDA) investigated the effects of several spices reported to improve diabetes, they were surprised that cinnamon, cloves, tumeric (mustard), and bay leaves actually had a measurable impact on making insulin more effective in the body. Of all these therapeutic herbs, cinnamon was the champion. Since cinnamon has no calories, makes insulin more effective, and makes food taste better, use it liberally.

ONION

Onions, whether cooked or raw, contain a substance, allyl propyl disulfide (APDS), that dramatically lowers blood sugar. APDS apparently helps to prevent the liver's

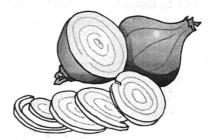

deactivation of insulin, which allows insulin to stay in the bloodstream longer and lower blood glucose. Onions actually came close to having the same therapeutic effect as the drug tolbutamide in animal studies. Eat onions often. Eat any color of onions, cooked or raw.

GARLIC

Garlic may be one of the more valuable foods on the planet earth for reversing both diabetes and the many complications of diabetes. First mentioned as a medicine about 6000 years ago, garlic has been a major player in human medicines throughout the world. In the tomb of the Egyptian

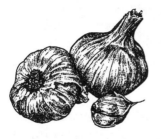

king, Tutankhamen, were found gold ornaments and garlic bulbs. Slaves who built the Great Pyramids relied heavily on the energizing power of garlic for their work. Hippocrates, father of modern medicine, used garlic to heal infections and reduce pain.

Although garlic has been a medical staple of many societies for over 4000 years, only in the past few decades when over 2000 scientific studies have proven its healing value, has garlic received the respect and attention that it deserves.

The debate continues regarding the active ingredients in garlic, but they may include amino acids (like the branched chain amino acids of leucine and isoleucine), S-allyl cysteine, allicin, and organically-bound selenium. In a double blind trial in humans with high serum cholesterol, aged deodorized garlic with no allicin content was able to lower serum cholesterol by 7%.[5] While garlic, in general as either aged, fresh, cooked or in supplement form, is a healthy addition to anyone's nutrition program; aged garlic extracts were effective at protecting animals from liver damage.[6]

Garlic helps to modify extremes in blood glucose. A study published in the Journal of the National Medical Association referred to garlic as "...a potent, non-specific biologic response modifier."[7] See the recipe section for fabulous microwave oven roasted garlic cloves.

GRAPEFRUIT

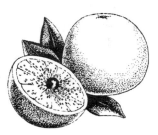

Since heart disease and cholesterol build up in the arteries is a prime enemy of the diabetic, grapefruit can come to the rescue. Dr. James Cerda, professor of gastroenterology at the University of Florida has found that the fiber in grapefruit can measurably lower serum cholesterol in humans. This fiber is not found in grapefruit juice, and less of it is found in the sectioned grapefruit that many Americans eat. Try quartering a whole grapefruit, then peel it, the cut out the center seed section with a sharp knife, then eat the remaining whole grapefruit as if it were a large tart orange. Delicious and good for you. Red grapefruit is also rich in bioflavonoids and carotenoids. Grapefruit is one of the best of all fruits for avoiding sharp rises in blood glucose.

SOLUBLE FIBER FOODS

Our ancestors consumed a diet containing 50 to 100 grams of fiber daily, with a rich mixture of both soluble and insoluble fibers. Today, we consume less than 20 grams of fiber, with a serious shortage of soluble fibers. This fundamental flaw in our diet along with too much sugar probably initiates more diabetes than any other nutrition factors mentioned in this book.

Soluble fiber forms a gelatinous mass in the fluid bath of the intestines, which creates an interfering net that slows down the absorption of glucose into the bloodstream. The following foods are rich sources of soluble fibers that can dramatically improve the course for Type 2 diabetes: brussel sprouts, okra, peas, broccoli, carrots, oat, beans, peas, garbanzo beans, sea vegetables.

PATIENT PROFILE

A.R. had watched her mother go through the various complications of uncontrolled diabetes, including blindness and kidney failure. A.R. vowed never to go through such an ordeal. But A.R. was diagnosed with Type 1 diabetes after she underwent a hysterectomy for a benign growth on her ovaries. The first year after her diagnosis she ate out of depression. Her weight and blood glucose levels went up and her physical and mental energy levels went down. When she came to me she was in tears for the fear of going through what her mother had experienced. I assured her that she could do a much better job of controlling her blood glucose through diet, exercise, weight loss, and supplements. She started using a teaspoon of brewer's yeast each morning in her pureed vegetable drink. She also took the high doses of niacin mentioned in the supplement chapter. Six months into her program, A.R. called me because she had a date, her first since her divorce 5 years ago. She looked, felt great, and had lost the need for insulin!!

ENDNOTES

[1]. Feskens, EJM, et al., Diabetes, Care, vol.14, p.935, 1991

[2]. Axelrod, L., Diabetes Care, vol.17, p.37, 1994

[3]. Brand-Miller, J., et al., THE GLUCOSE REVOLUTION, p.43, Marlowe & Co., NYC, 1999

[4]. Schmidt, MA, SMART FATS, p.9, Frog Ltd, Berkeley, 1997

[5]. Steiner, M., et al., Amer.J.Clin.Nutr., vol.64, p.866, 1996

[6]. Nakagawa, S., et al., Phytotherapy Res., vol.1, p.1, 1988

[7]. Abdullah, TH, et al., J.Nat.Med.Assoc., vol.80, p.439, 1988

CHAPTER 7

SWEETENERS

THE GOOD, THE BAD, AND THE UGLY

"The people think the FDA is protecting them--it isn't. What the FDA is doing and what the public thinks it's doing are as different as night and day." Former FDA Commissioner Dr. Herbert L. Ley, 1969

Wandering the streets of many different towns in Mexico, I was appalled at the number of people with bad teeth, all of whom were drinking colas and chewing gum. Rotting or silver or gold teeth are almost universal in many underdeveloped countries. A friend of mine who has visited the remote areas of Bolivia says the same thing. As soon as third world people have any disposable income, they spend much of their money on sugary foods which rot their teeth. Mothers would provide cola in baby bottles for their infants, with the resulting infant growing baby teeth already full of cavities. These same people then begin the cycle of developing the "diseases of civilization". This chapter is about making good decisions when it comes to chosing sweeteners to use on your food.

Sugar makes food taste good. Mother's milk is sweet. Fresh fruit is sweet. The Old Testament is full of references to the wonder of sweets.

"So I have come down to rescue them from the hand of the Egyptians and to bring them up out of that land into a good and spacious land, a land flowing with milk and honey" Exodus 3:8

A special region of our tongue is exclusively reserved for finding and appreciating sweet foods. This makes good sense. Sweet foods are more likely to have carbohydrates for nourishment and less likely to be poisonous, such as some bitter plants. Our hunter-gatherer ancestors were hard pressed

Sugar consumption in America: pounds/person/year

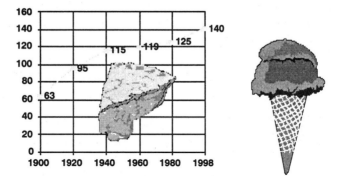

source: American J. Health Promotion, 11:42, 1996

to find sweet foods, and thus their bodies were forced to make glucose out of proteins in the body. However, once mankind developed the technology for growing and concentrating refined sugars in unimaginable levels, that sweet tooth of ours has become our enemy within. That sweet tooth leads us on to greater and greater heights of sugar intake like a moth drawn to a flame.

My first recommendation in chosing a sweetener for your food is to cut back dramatically on total sweetener intake: either caloric or non-caloric. By doing so, you will begin to taste the flavors of the food and begin to lose that sweetness craving. Once you have cut back your intake of caloric sugars from the current average of 140 pounds per year per person to a more reasonable 50 pounds per year and have removed all aspartame (NutraSweet) from your diet, then choose from the preferred sweeteners listed below.

The alphabet of sugars:
Disaccharide means 2 sugar molecules together, like table sugar, or sucrose.
Monosaccharide means 1 sugar molecule, like fructose in honey or fruits.
glucose + fructose=sucrose (table sugar)
glucose + glucose=maltose
glucose + galactose=lactose (milk sugar)

CALORIC SWEETENERS
contain 4 kcal per gram & can cause cavities
SUGAR: Based upon federal laws passed after World War II to protect the California and Hawaii sugar industry, a "sugar" must have at least 96% of all other plant matter stripped from it in order to be called sugar. 90% of the bulk of cane sugar is fiber, protein, and other matter. All of this is lost in the sugar refining process. Therefore, turbinado sugar, brown sugar and other health food store sugars are virtually identical to white sugar in nutrient density and glycemic index.

Barley malt is a mild natural sweetener made from barley sprouts that is less sweet and less hazardous on blood glucose levels than other sweeteners listed here, yet very expensive.

Blackstrap molasses: What's left over at the bottom of the barrel from the sugar refining industry. Molasses contains the concentrated vitamins and minerals that were once in the cane sugar, though it still can create havoc with blood glucose levels and has an unusual wild taste. Has more calcium than milk, more iron than eggs, and a rich source of potassium.

Brown sugar: can be made by blending white sugar with molasses. Little advantage over white sugar.

Corn syrup is commercial glucose from cornstarch with some sucrose syrup added. Very refined food with a very high glycemic index.

Date sugar is ground and dried dates from desert climates. Tasty whole food, but high glycemic index.

⇒Fructose is found in many fruits, honey and as pure crystalline fructose, is slowly absorbed in the intestinal tract, and requires the liver to convert fructose to glucose for body use. Glycemic index of 20. Very useful for diabetics.

Fruit juice concentrate is usually made from grape juice and, due to a high fructose concentration, has a favorable glycemic index.

Glucose/dextrose: Here is the gold currency of sugar in the blood. Glucose is usually extracted from corn syrup and is rapidly absorbed from the intestines into the bloodstream. Foods high in glucose (watermelon, parsnips) or starches easily digested into glucose (like rice cakes or white bread) can create rapid and dangerous rises in blood glucose.

Gymnema sylvestre is a valuable herb discussed in more detail in the "supplement" chapter. I mention it here because it can block the taste of sugar in the mouth. Using gymnema tea with those occasional sweet snacks can help to reduce the amount of sugar that you crave.

Honey is formed when bees partially digest nectar from flowers. Honey has well documented value as an antiseptic, antibiotic, and stomach calming food. Honey from your nearby vicinity can help with allergies and is a real food vs. the "cadaver" state of most other highly refined caloric sweeteners. Honey varies in taste and content based on the hives and flowers in your region. Honey is usually about 31% glucose, 38% fructose, 18% water, 9% other sugars, and 2% sucrose. Yet, honey, in excess, can create problems with glycemic index and weight.

Lactose (milk sugar). About 50-90% of adults are lactose intolerant and therefore do not digest this sugar well, which then generates intestinal cramps, constipation, gas, or diarrhea. In yogurt, the lactose has been fermented by healthy bacteria into lactic acid, hence the slightly tart taste. People who are lactose intolerant can usually consume yogurt with no problem.

Maltitol is a relatively new sugar found in health food stores. Made from corn, maltitol has a better glycemic index than sucrose and 25% fewer calories per gram. However, it is expensive and not as sweet as table sugar.

Maple syrup is concentrated sweetener from the sap of sugar maple trees. It requires 30-40 gallons of sap to make 1 gallon of maple syrup. Unless the product is labelled "pure" maple syrup, then it is probably diluted with corn syrup to cut the cost. Though the flavor is unique, the glycemic index is little better than white sugar.

Rice syrup is made by culturing rice with digestive enzymes to break down the starch into glucose. Tasty whole food, but high glycemic index.

Sorghum molasses is the concentrated juice from the sorghum plant, a cereal grain. Has a lighter flavor than blackstrap molasses.

Sucanat: trade name that means "SUgar CAne NATural" and comes from ground up organically grown sugar cane. 85% is sugar, with the balance of 15% being fiber, vitamins, minerals, amino acids, and molasses. Though Sucanat is a whole food, it is more expensive and provides a minor advantage in nutrient density and glycemic index vs white table sugar.

Sucrose is basic table sugar and merits a special discussion here. It was around 600 AD that Persians began growing and refining sugar cane into something similar to our white table sugar. Since then, sugar has been a pivotal point in history, wars, taxes, and even the Declaration of Independence of the United States of America. The immoral trade route that connected the continents of Europe, Africa, and North America for centuries involved buying slaves from Africa with rum to sell the slaves to sugar cane plantations in the Caribbean, then bring the sugar, molasses, and rum to Europe and Africa for more trade. Long before the Boston Tea Party, the Molasses Act of 1733 put British rule in the crosshairs of American colonists. At the time of the revolutionary war, the average annual consumption of molasses rum was 4 gallons per man, woman, and child. One could argue that the enthusiastic consumption of sugar and its by-products have been instrumental in bringing us the "diseases of civilization", including tuberculosis, diabetes, heart disease, many forms of cancer (which is a sugar-feeder), various mental disorders (including hyperactivity), and more. Suffice it to say that sucrose is more of a drug than a food. Consume it with all due caution.

Turbinado sugar is raw sugar that has been washed of its molasses content in a centrifuge. Basically, it is overpriced white sugar.

CALORIC BUT NON-CARIOGENIC
contain 4 kcal per gram and cannot cause cavities

Sorbitol is derived from corn, absorbed slowly, requires little insulin, and is used in many foods for diabetics. Probably safe, but may cause diarrhea in some sensitive individuals. Use in moderation.

Xylitol is extracted from birchwood chips and used in chewing gum. May reduce cavities by neutralizing the acids in the mouth. Use in moderation.

NON-CALORIC SWEETENERS
no calories & no cavities

⇒Stevia, or stevioside, is extracted from a sweetening herb, stevia rebaudiana, and does not have either calories or a long and checkered past like many of the other artificial sweeteners listed here. Stevia was commercialized in the 1970s by a Japanese firm and still enjoys over 40% of the food sweetener market in both South America and Asia. Stevia has been used as a natural sweetener for over 1500 years in South America. The herb is actually beneficial for people with poorly regulated blood glucose, though the concentrated extract, stevioside sold in health food stores, does not retain these healing properties. The FDA created a bizarre and suspicious import ban on stevia for years, which was recently lifted. Stevioside and stevia are the safest and most recommended of the artificial sweeteners available today.

Splenda, or sucralose, is a relatively new artificial sweetener invented in 1976, patented by a subsidiary of Johnson & Johnson, and approved by the Food and Drug Administration in 1998. Splenda is made from sugar, is stable in cooking, tastes like sugar, but cannot cause dental caries and does not raise blood sugar. Splenda has a molecule that is slightly different in shape from normal table sugar and has a chlorine atom added. Splenda is in such great demand that it is only available from the Johnson & Johnson internet website (www.sucralose.com) for adult diabetics. Other interested consumers will have to wait until production can meet the demand. Preliminary evidence indicates that Splenda is relatively safe, especially compared to aspartame.

✖ Aspartame provides us with a classical example of how the FDA is not protecting the American consumer, but rather creating extremely profitable monopolies for those who can afford the $150 million investment required to pass the "safety tests". Aspartame, Equal or NutraSweet (trademark of the NutraSweet Company) is consumed by over 100 million people in the US alone. It is 180 times sweeter than table sugar, is included in over 1200 products in America, and was approved by the FDA in 1981. Over a billion pounds of aspartame are used annually in the US. I will spare you the detailed accounts of how aspartame has been linked to our 250% rise in brain cancer since its approval[1], or the double blind study by psychiatrists that was halted because aspartame created such blatant depression in the test subjects[2], or the study showing that aspartame caused headaches in a double blind trial[3], or the fact that of the 2800 FDA approved food additives, 80% of all complaints are regarding aspartame.[4] Aspartame breaks down after long term storage, heating, and in the body into wood alcohol (methyl alcohol) and dangerous isomers of the amino acid phenylalanine. Researcher Richard Wurtman, MD of MIT cautioned the FDA on the approval of aspartame, noting the rise in brain tumors among animals fed aspartame. Along with the meteoric rise in the consumption of aspartame has come a parallel rise in the incidence of both obesity and morbid obesity (people who are dangerously overweight). I strongly discourage the use of aspartame. I would rather have a diabetic judiciously use white table sugar than use aspartame.

Saccharin is a chemical derivative of petroleum and toluene, a solvent used to reduce the knocking in automobile engines.[5] Saccharin was found to increase the incidence of bladder cancer in animals, but under pressure from lobbyists, the FDA allowed saccharin to remain on the market with a warning label. I discourage the use of saccharin, but consider it safer than aspartame.

PATIENT PROFILE

T.M. was a truck driver who lived on fast food, gravy, and beer. When he started having to stop often to go to the bathroom while driving his big rig, he thought something might be very wrong. His doctor found his blood glucose levels to be around 400 mg%, yet his insulin levels were adequate. He told me that he would make some compromises in the dietary department if I could suggest some nutrition supplements that would help bring down his blood glucose. I suggested 400 mg of magnesium, 400 mcg of chromium picolinate, 200 mg Gymnema sylvestre herb, and a few other nutrients, like vitamin E and C. His diet improved, but was far from "pristine" in the no fat/no sugar categories. Yet, his blood glucose went down to fasting levels of 100-150 mg%. A major improvement which allowed him to get back on the road. His wife of 27 years was pleased to see his better health and have him back on the road again, since he had tried to rearrange her entire kitchen while he was home.

ENDNOTES

[1] . Olney, JW, et al., J.Neuropathol.Exp.Neurol., vol.55, p.1115, 1996

[2] . Walton, RG, et al., Biol.Psychiatry, vol.34, p.13, 1993

[3] . VanDen Eeden, SK, et al., Neurology, vol.44, p.1787, Oct.1994

[4] . Roberts, HJ, ASPARTAME: IS IT SAFE?, p.12, Charles Press, Philadelphia, 1990

[5] . Page, LR, HEALTHY HEALING, p.199, Healthy Healing Publ, 1996

CHAPTER 8

NUTRITION SUPPLEMENTS
TO IMPROVE DIABETES

VITAMINS ARE ESSENTIAL FOR DIABETICS

"In the US, the incidence of diabetes has increased proportionately with the per capita consumption of sugar. In the heating and recrystallization of the natural sugar cane, something is altered which leaves the refined product a dangerous foodstuff." Dr. Frederick Banting, Nobel prize winner, discoverer of insulin, 1929

There are now over 20,000 scientific studies showing the benefits of nutrition supplements in humans. Concentrated pills, powders, and tinctures of vitamins, minerals, herbs, fatty acids, glandulars, food extracts, and homeopathic preparations can go a long way toward bringing the diabetic out of a "survival" poor health status and moving toward a "thriving" health status.

Many doctors still parrot the old adage about supplements: "If you just eat a good diet, then you don't need them." Yet the Standard American Diet (SAD) consists of 60% of the calories from nutrient depleted fat and sugar. Based on government surveys, 92% of all Americans do not get the RDA for all essential nutrients. And, as you will read in this chapter, diabetics have an elevated need for various nutrients.

Nutrition supplements have moved from a controversial status in the 1980s to a very respectable status in the 1990s. However, the official position of most governmental agencies, like the Food and Drug Administration is basically: "If you eat a good diet, then you don't need nutrition supplements. And furthermore, if nutrition supplements actually have a therapeutic benefit, then they should be regulated by the FDA and a physician's prescription." Fortunately, the Congressional Dietary Supplement Health and Education Act (DSHEA) of 1994 mandated that the FDA must not restrict access to supplements unless the FDA can prove that they are harmful. And supplements are extremely safe, especially when compared to the likelihood of the diabetic developing some disastrous complication as a result of not having enough of some nutrient.

NUTRITION SUPPLEMENTS ARE SAFE

While 400,000 Americans die each year as a consequence of tobacco use, and another 125,000 die from the side effects of using prescription medication, there have been NO DEATHS from the use of nutrition supplements in the past 5 years. Since 17 Americans die each year from electrocution while using a hair dryer in the bathtub, nutrition supplements are much safer than almost any risk faced by Americans.

The following data was reported in the New York Academy of Sciences textbook MICRONUTRIENTS AND IMMUNE FUNCTION (vol.587, p.257, 1990) by John Hathcock, PhD, a Food and Drug Administration toxicologist,

>Vitamin A toxicity may start as low as 25,000 iu/day (5 times RDA) in people with impaired liver function via drugs, hepatitis, or protein malnutrition. Otherwise, toxicity for A begins at several hundred thousand iu/day.

>Beta-carotene given at 180 mg/day (300,000 iu or 60 times RDA) for extended periods produced no toxicity, but mild carotenemia (orange pigmentation of skin).

>Vitamin E at 300 iu/day (10 times RDA) can trigger nausea, fatigue, and headaches in sensitive individuals. Otherwise, few side effects are seen at up to 3,200 iu/day.

>B-6 may induce a reversible sensory neuropathy at doses of as low as 300 mg/day in some sensitive individuals. Toxic threshold usually begins at 2000 mg for most individuals.

>Vitamin C may induce mild and transient gastro-intestinal distress in some sensitive individuals at doses of 1000 mg (16 times RDA). Otherwise, toxicity is very rare at even high doses of vitamin C intake.

>Zinc supplements at 300 mg (20 times RDA) have been found to impair immune functions and serum lipid profile.

>Iron intake at 100 mg/day (6 times RDA) will cause iron storage disease in 80% of population. The "window of efficacy" on iron is probably more narrow than with other nutrients.

>Copper can be toxic, though dose is probably related to the ratio with other trace minerals.

>Selenium can be toxic at 1-5 mg/kg body weight intake. This would equate to 65 mg/day for the average adult, which is 812 times the RDA of 80 mcg. Some sensitive individuals may develop toxicity at 1000 mcg/day.

>Manganese can be toxic, though little specific information can be provided for humans.

The bottom line is: Nutrition supplements are very safe, especially at the dosages mentioned in this chapter. While normal healthy adults who eat an excellent diet probably can get along without nutrition supplements, diabetics need supplements even if they are eating a very good diet.

You may wish to purchase any or all of the following supplements either at your local health food store or through the many mail order companies listed in the back appendix.

FIBER 40-50 GRAMS/DAY

Based upon a huge amount of human and animal studies, it could be that diabetes is more related to a deficiency of dietary fiber than any other nutrition substance.[1] Fiber is indigestible plant food matter. Because fiber cannot be digested in the human gut, it stays in the intestines to slow down the absorption of glucose into the bloodstream, while it simultaneously absorbs excess fat and cholesterol to carry these potential trouble makers out of the system.

There are two main types of fiber: soluble (in water) and insoluble. Soluble fibers form a gelatin-like mass in the intestines. Examples of soluble fibers include hemicelluloses, mucilages, gums, and pectins; such as found in apples, carrots, oats, and beans. Insoluble fibers can help with other conditions, such as weight loss, but are not as helpful in slowing down the absorption of glucose to control diabetes. Dr. James Anderson at the University of Kentucky has spent 2 decades studying the various dietary approaches to Type 2 diabetes that can be of the most benefit. A diet rich in soluble fiber and legumes improves all aspects of diabetes.[2] For example, Dr. David Jenkins, the developer of the glycemic index chart, found that diabetics who consumed between 14 to 26 grams of guar gum soluble fiber required less insulin and had better control of their blood glucose levels.[3]

Consume around 50 grams of fiber daily, which is a 250% increase over the standard low fiber American diet. In addition to the many foods which contribute significant amounts of soluble fiber to the diabetic diet, nutrition supplements found in your health food store include: glucomannan, guar gum, oat gum, pea fiber, pectin, and psyllium. Some remarkably useful nutrition supplements in this category include Perfect 7 (714-229-8866).

VITAMINS

VITAMIN C 500-2000 MG/DAY

Vitamin C is a molecule that looks very similar to glucose. Not surprisingly, it requires insulin to get vitamin C into most body cells. Also, a high intake of vitamin C can create abnormal readings on everything from urine to blood glucose measurements. So, be aware that supplements of vitamin C can reduce complications in diabetes, but may increase the chances for false readings of body sugar levels in both blood and urine.

Most diabetics have a deficiency of vitamin C in spite of consuming the Recommended Dietary Allowance (RDA) level.[4] This deficiency of vitamin C will oftentimes lead to symptoms of scurvy: reduced immunity against infections and increased tendency to bleed from capillary permeability, poor wound healing, vascular disease, and high cholesterol. Supplements of 2000 milligrams daily of vitamin C in human diabetics has been shown to slow down the "tanning" or glycosylation of proteins in the blood, while also helping the body to avoid the toxic accumulation of sorbitol inside the cells.[5] Because of the serious toxicity of sorbitol buildup in the diabetic cells, pharmaceutical companies have developed a drug to help purge sorbitol from the cells (aldose reductase inhibitors), yet in a clinical trial vitamin C was superior to the drug at both reducing sorbitol in the cells and being without side effects.

NIACIN (B-3) 500-1000 MG/DAY

Niacin is a key nutrient in the burning of calories as well as the making of the Glucose Tolerance Factor that helps insulin move glucose through the cell membrane. The best tolerated form of niacin in the reduction of diabetic complications is inositol hexaniacinate, which has been helpful both in reducing fats in the blood for all diabetics and sometimes even reversing early onset Type 1 diabetes. Yes, you read that correctly. It used to be thought that once the pancreas had been destroyed and Type 1diabetes sets in, that person will forever be an insulin dependent diabetic. Yet 10 studies have investigated the value of niacin supplements to help reverse early onset Type 1 diabetes. Most of these studies have shown a positive result in lowering insulin requirements, improved pancreatic beta cell function, and overall enhancement of blood glucose regulation. In the patients who received a complete remission--their Type 1 diabetes was cured--those most likely to get this gift were older and had more pancreatic function (based on fasting C-peptide in the blood).[6] It seems that in younger people who have had destruction of the beta cells of the pancreas, the auto-immune attack is so swift and merciless, that little is left of the pancreas to resurrect.

Type 2 diabetics using 1800 mg to 3000 mg of inositol hexaniacinate daily had an average of 18% reduction in total cholesterol, 26% reduction in triglycerides, and 30% increase in the heart protective HDL cholesterol.

BIOTIN 9 MG/DAY

Biotin is a B-vitamin that is very involved in energy metabolism. Biotin supplements increase insulin sensitivity, while also increasing the activity of a liver enzyme (glucokinase) that helps the body metabolize glucose. In a study of Type 1 diabetics, 16 mg/day of biotin significantly lowered fasting blood glucose levels and improved overall blood glucose control. Type 2 diabetics received equally impressive results using 9 mg/day of biotin.[7] Biotin supplements must be mentioned to your physician, because diabetics typically can sometimes lower their medication requirements by using biotin. Biotin is one of the more expensive of all vitamins.

B-6 (PYRIDOXINE) 50-100 MG

Vitamin B-6 is crucial for the manufacturing of insulin and the production of all proteins in the body. Supplements of B-6 have been very effective at slowing and reversing the neuropathies found in many diabetics.[8] B-6 also prevents the glycosylation, or "tanning", of proteins that occurs when too much glucose is lingering in the bloodstream. In a study with 14 women with gestational diabetes , 100 mg/day of B-6 cured 12 (85%) of the subjects.[9]

B-12:   300-3000 MCG/DAY

Vitamin B-12 (along with folacin) is involved in new cell growth. The deficiency symptoms of B-12 include numbness of the feet, tingling and burning sensation, "pins and needles" feeling--which are the same sensations of diabetic neuropathy. Supplements of B-12 have had some success in reversing neuropathy[10] and retinopathy in diabetics.[11] No one knows whether these super high levels (300 times the RDA) are correcting imbalances in the cells of diabetics or filling in deficiencies.

E (D-ALPHA TOCOPHEROL) 400-2000 MG/DAY

Vitamin E is the primary fat soluble antioxidant in the bloodstream. Since diabetics are prone toward excess levels of "rusting", or oxidized, fats in the blood and 80% of diabetics die from heart disease, vitamin E can become a valuable shield in the storm of free radicals being generated in the body of the diabetic patient. Remember, the insulin receptors on the cell membrane are made from fats, which are rusting at a higher rate in diabetics.

In one study 10 healthy controls and 15 Type 2 diabetics took 1350 IU (international units) of vitamin E daily with substantial improvements in ALL subjects, especially the diabetics, in glucose metabolism and insulin action.[12] Vitamin E may also prevent diabetes. One study followed 944 men, ages 42-60, for four years. 45 of these men developed diabetes. Those men who had the lowest levels of vitamin E in the blood had a 400% increase in the risk of developing Type 2 diabetes.[13]

MINERALS

CHROMIUM 200-800 MICROGRAMS

Long ago, our ancestors would fertilize their fields with compost and manure. This "full spectrum" fertilization concept kept trace minerals, like chromium, in the soil and in the food supply. Today, modern agri-business does not add chromium to the soil and, hence, each time we harvest a crop, there is proportionately less amounts of chromium both in the soil and

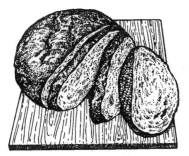

the food supply. We then take what precious chromium is in the food and strip it out in the milling of grains and the refining of sugar. While the Food and Nutrition Board of the National Academy of Sciences considers 50-200 micrograms daily of chromium to be adequate, 90% of Americans do not consume at least 50 mcg of chromium per day.

Chromium plays a pivotal role in the crucial molecule "Glucose Tolerance Factor" which, along with insulin, "opens the doors" of the cell membrane to allow glucose into the cell for fuel. Chromium deficiency is common in America, even by conservative standards, and plays a major role in the growing incidence of Type 2 diabetes in this country.[14] Chromium supplements seem to benefit diabetics who are chromium deficient, which is the majority.

In one large placebo-controlled trial examining the role of chromium supplements in Type 2 diabetes, 60 diabetics were given placebo (inert ingredients), 60 others were given 200 mcg of chromium daily, and the third group of 60 diabetics were given 1000 mcg of chromium daily. All patients continued their medication and medical monitoring of their condition. Chromium supplements helped regulate fasting glucose, reduce glycosylated hemoglobin, insulin values and total cholesterol--all in a dose-dependent fashion, meaning that 1000 mcg of chromium worked better than the 200 mcg dosage.

Best food sources of chromium are foods grown on chromium rich soil, which is a "hit or miss" concept because most of us don't know where our food is grown. Liver, meat, cheese, legumes, beans, peas, whole grains and molasses (but not white flour or white sugar) are good sources of chromium. Far and away the richest source of the active form of chromium, Glucose Tolerance Factor, is brewer's yeast. See the "superfood" chapter.

MAGNESIUM 300-600 MG

The body is a rich soup of minerals with one of the more important and multi-talented minerals being magnesium. Magnesium is involved in each of the trillions of energy reactions that occur daily to generate ATP in the body as well as nerve and muscle function. Low intake of magnesium is a major risk factor in the deterioration of diabetic complications, especially retinopathy.[15]

The RDA for magnesium for males is 350 milligrams daily. Twice that amount (750 mg) would be a good target for diabetics. The average American consumes 143-266 mg daily of magnesium due to our highly refined food supply. Best food sources of magnesium are soy, legumes, seeds, nuts, whole grains, and green leafy vegetables. For an inexpensive magnesium supplement, take 1/4 to 1/2 teaspoon of food grade

(USP) Epsom salts (magnesium sulfate) from your pharmacy. Cost is less than a penny per day.

POTASSIUM 5-6 GRAMS

With sodium being the primary mineral outside of all cell membranes, potassium is the major mineral inside all cell membranes. The electrical charge from these minerals generates what is called "membrane potential" or the energy that constitutes the batteries in each of our cells. One of the primary theories about why Type 2 diabetics develop insulin resistance is that the sodium/potassium membrane potential in the cell is off kilter, leading to insulin not being able to open the doors in the cell membrane.

A high potassium diet has been shown to lower the risk for diabetes, cancer, heart disease, and improves glucose tolerance. Plant foods like fruits, vegetables, whole grains, and legumes, are the best sources of potassium. Potassium supplements are regulated by the FDA, since excess potassium can become hazardous for the ailing kidneys of advanced diabetic patients. Potassium supplements in diabetics with healthy kidneys can come from physician prescription or by using salt substitutes, which are potassium chloride. CAUTION: advised in diabetics with kidney complications

SULFUR (METHYL SULFONYL METHANE)

Sulfur is one of the most important yet ignored minerals in human nutrition. While the average human body has 6 times more sulfur than magnesium, most nutrition textbooks only give brief and passing reference to sulfur.[16] Sulfur is your "steel rebar" in structural proteins in the body, which is why there is more sulfur in a meat eater's diet of flesh than a vegetarian diet. Sulfur is also a crucial mineral for detoxification and improving cell membrane permeability. Most agri-businesses ignore the need to fertilize the soil with sulfur, hence each time we harvest the crops, we have

progressively less sulfur in our food supply.
Methylsulfonylmethane, or MSM, is an organically bound form
of sulfur which is better for your body. Inorganic forms of
sulfur, such as the preservative sulfites found in dried fruit and
wine can be harmful and do not contribute to the body's need
for organically bound sulfur.

Algae and phytoplankton in the ocean and ponds
everywhere take in inorganic sulfur and release a volatile
vapor, dimethyl sulfide, which rises in the atmosphere and is
converted into DMSO by the action of the sun's ultra-violet
light. Add an oxygen atom to DMSO and you have DMSO2,
which is MSM.[17] These sulfur-bearing compounds then mix
with rain clouds and scatter over the world to provide organic
sulfur for plants. On an ecological note, sulfites and sulfates
from cars and factories can react in the atmosphere to form
sulfuric acid, which makes acid rain that has been devastating
forests around the world.

MSM is found in small amounts in fresh plant foods,
but is easily lost in storage, cooking, and processing. Hence,
most of us get very little MSM in the diet. MSM has the health
advantages of DMSO without giving the user the characteristic
"garlic breath" that is almost immediately apparent when
rubbing DMSO on the skin. MSM is very safe, since it is
found in small amounts in fresh produce and is, therefore,
either used or excreted by the body. Since MSM is a patented
compound, it is referred to in scientific literature as "polar
solvents" or "dimethyl sulfone".

Sulfur is a critical ingredient in some of the healthiest
foods on earth: garlic, beans, eggs, cabbage, broccoli, and red
peppers. Sulfur used to be called "brimstone", and was a threat
of sorts from the "fire and brimstone" preachers of old.
Flowers of sulfur is a yellow powder that our grandparents
would sometimes sprinkle in their shoes to help ward off
rheumatoid arthritis.

MSM may help diabetic patients in the following ways:
- ♥ Blood glucose regulation. Insulin contains several sulfur atoms to give it a unique three dimensional shape and function in regulating blood glucose. People who are deficient in sulfur will probably develop diabetic-like symptoms.
- ♥ Regular bowel movements. According to the "grandfather" of DMSO, Dr. Stanley Jacobs, MSM seems to induce regularity and treat constipation without side effects.[18]
- ♥ Immune regulation. There is some evidence that DMSO and its metabolite, dimethyl sulfone, may help to downregulate an over reactive immune system in autoimmune diseases.[19]
- ♥ Membrane fluidity. Since sulfur is a crucial component of every cell membrane in every form of life on earth, some experts have speculated that low intake of sulfur can lead to defective cell membrane functions. Cell membranes are the "gate keepers", with the assignment of expelling toxins and bringing in essential nutrients. If the cell membrane fails in either the intake or output processes, we can have a cell that begins to reject insulin or glucose and begins the slide down the slippery slope of diabetes.

MANGANESE

Manganese deficient animals develop low insulin output, problems with the connective tissue and processing of fats. Recommended intake is 2-5 milligrams daily for adults, with over half the female population consuming less than adequate amounts of manganese.[20] Best food sources of manganese are whole grains, nuts and fruits grown on manganese rich (properly fertilized) soil. There are at least 3 different minerals, including manganese, copper, and zinc, that play a role in variations of the critical antioxidant enzyme system SOD.

ZINC 10-60 MG/DAY

Zinc is the most multi-talented mineral in the body, participating in everything from sexual development, to immunity, to maintenance of nerve tissue, to the zinc-dependent antioxidant enzyme SOD (superoxide dismutase). The average American consumes about 10 milligrams of zinc daily, which is well shy of the 15 mg RDA. Best food sources of zinc include shell fish, organ meats, meat, fish, pumpkin seeds, ginger root, nuts and seeds.

Zinc is a crucial mineral for optimal immune functioning. Reduced zinc levels and diabetes are both common in the elderly. Loss of appetite is one of the first symptoms of zinc deficiency

SAFETY ISSUES. Supplements of zinc should be in the 10-60 mg/day range, since doses of 150 mg/day have been shown to trigger copper deficiency and depress the cardio-protective HDL-cholesterol.

VANADIUM

Vanadium is not added back to the soil in agri-business, and hence may be missing from the American diet, which typically contains 10-60 micrograms daily of vanadium.[21] When non-insulin dependent diabetics were supplemented with 100 milligrams daily (100,000 micrograms) of vanadyl sulfate, blood glucose levels dropped by 14%.[22] Vanadium in the form of vanadyl sulfate has shown promise in helping to control rises in blood glucose in human diabetics.[23] Toxicity may begin at 13 milligrams (13,000 micrograms) of vanadium daily. Best food sources of vanadium include mushrooms, shellfish, dill, parsley and black pepper.

ESSENTIAL FATTY ACIDS

FISH & FLAX

Not all fat is created equally. Fat-phobic Americans have lost sight of the fact that there are good, bad and ugly fats.

DIETARY FATS		
GOOD	**BAD**	**UGLY**
flax, olive, canola, fish, primrose, borage, MCT, lecithin, rice bran, rapeseed, hemp	too much fat of any kind, especially in a deficiency state of vitamin E (protects against fat "rusting")	hydrogenated (lard), or oxidized (from fast food deep fryers), or not enough vit.E or too much sugar

When the Senate Diet Goals were released by a blue ribbon panel of nutrition experts in 1977, they included the recommendation to decrease fat intake from 40% of calories to 30%. Yet, experts then looked at the Greenland Eskimos, who get 60% of their calories from fat and practically no dietary fiber, yet mysteriously had no diabetes, cancer, or heart disease. Three factors saved these people from an otherwise disastrous diet:

1) genetic adaption, at least 40,000 years to adjust to this uniquely skewed diet

2) fish oil, which contains a very special and highly unsaturated fat, eicosapentaenoic acid, or EPA for short.

3) no sugar in the diet, which helps the body make PGE-1, a healthy prostaglandin

EPA is, essentially, Nature's anti-freeze. In the arctic regions of the world, the ocean temperature drops to below freezing, yet water-based life will explode at that temperature, like leaving out a water balloon on a sub-freezing night. So Nature provides the algae in the ocean with this special fat,

EPA, that prevents freezing and bursting at low temperatures. Smaller fish eat the algae, and bigger fish eat the smaller fish, until we have major concentrations of EPA in cold water fish, like cod, salmon, mackeral, tuna, and sardines. Much of the fat in seals and whales that were consumed by the Greenland Eskimos was rich in EPA, which provided these people with extraordinary protection against many diseases.

EPA may help the diabetic patient:

⇒**Changes membrane fluidity.** Cell membranes contain fats which are a direct reflection from our diet, including the unnatural hydrogenated fats found in Crisco and Pop Tarts. When we are talking about dietary fats, the old saying is literally true, "you are what you eat." Cell membranes that are fluid, flexible and allow the proper nutrients, like glucose, to pass into the cell will improve overall wellness. Cells that are flexible with EPA can squeeze down narrow capillaries to feed the distant tissue. Cells that are rigid with too much saturated or hydrogenated fat or having been "tanned" from too much sugar in the blood will not be able to move down narrow capillaries, like a car trying to get down a hotel hallway.

⇒**Increase prostaglandin E-1**, a.k.a. PGE-1, which favors reducing the stickiness of cells for less risk of heart disease or stroke. PGE-1 also bolsters immune functions, dilates blood vessels, and elevates production of estrogen receptors.

BORAGE AND EVENING PRIMROSE

Our ancestors consumed a diet of range fed animals who grazed on wild grain, nuts and seeds. In these foods is a wide assortment of valuable fatty acids, including gamma linolenic acid (GLA), which is richly concentrated in the evening primrose and borage plants. Intake of GLA in modern Americans has dropped off substantially with the consumption of corn-fed beef, which is rich in linoleic acid that generates the tumor-promoting eicosanoid of arachidonic acid. The reason why range-fed lean buffalo was good for Native Americans, yet corn-fed high fat beef is not so good for modern Americans is primarily the quality and quantity of fats in these two animals. A ratio of approximately 4:1 of EPA to GLA is very favorable for making cell membranes that accept insulin and glucose in healthy fashion. Diabetics probably lose the ability to make optimal amounts of GLA in the body, which makes supplements essential.

We are able to make less GLA internally as we age, are exposed to stress and toxins, become compromised by disease, and eat hydrogenated fats--which describes millions of Americans. GLA in the diet helps to drive PGE-1, mentioned above, which is good.

CLA

Recently, I had to find a cable to connect my computer to my monitor. This was no easy task. In describing my needs to the salesperson, we got into a spirited discussion of how many pins in how many rows for each end of the cable. "Close" is not good enough in either computer cables or fatty acid requirements in the human body. Americans often consume fats that are unhealthy, like hydrogenated fats, and are deficient in valuable fats, like CLA. A tiny difference in molecular structure, just like computer cables, can make a huge difference in whether this fat will help or hinder your cellular machinery.

Conjugated linoleic acid, or CLA, is a collection of unique "18 pin" fatty acids found primarily in the meat and milk of grazing animals, like beef and dairy. CLA is one of the more exciting recent developments in therapeutic fats. There is 300-400% more CLA in spring and summer milk and most Australian dairy products due to the availability of fresh green pasture land, which augments CLA content in the milk and fat of grazing animals.[24]

CLA makes a good argument for humans consuming an omnivorous diet, since there is far more CLA, carnitine, EPA, taurine, and lipoic acid in animal foods than plants foods. Dr. Weston Price toured the world in the 1930s with his nurse-wife visiting numerous cultures and found many different diets--but he never found a group of people who were complete vegan. All of our ancestors ate some animal food. Maybe CLA is one of the nutrients that we need from a healthy mixed diet.

Bacteria in the gut of ruminants, like cows, sheep, deer and buffalo, can produce CLA. Yet there is more CLA in grilled beef than raw beef, so the cooking process also enhances CLA content.[25] CLA may be able to help the diabetic patient through:

♥ Improve glucose and insulin levels. CLA manages to also make cells more sensitive to insulin, thus lowering insulin requirements and blood glucose levels. These researchers from Penn State and Purdue boldly state: "CLA may prove to be an important therapy for the prevention and treatment of non-insulin dependent diabetes mellitus."[26]

♥ Antioxidant. There is a large and growing list of non-essential dietary antioxidants, including CLA, ellagic acid, curcumin, quercetin, and epicatechin, which have shown remarkable abilities to slow down the oxidative damage, or the "rusting" that occurs constantly in most diabetics. [27]

Basically, CLA is one of the more promising, non-toxic, inexpensive, anti-cancer, anti-heart disease, anti-diabetes nutrients to come along in the history of nutrition science.

QUASI-VITAMINS are nutrients that fall into a gray zone of nutrition, neither considered essential for survival by the National Academy of Sciences, nor considered in the "ignore" category based on good science. Diabetics may need quasi-vitamins in order to prevent or slow down the common complications of the disease.

LIPOIC ACID 100-500 MG

Lipoic acid works with pyruvate and acetyl CoA in a critical point in energy metabolism.[28] Partly because of this pivotal job in generating ATP, lipoic acid becomes an incredibly multi-talented nutrient. Though lipoic acid is not considered an essential nutrient yet, as humans age we produce less and less of lipoic acid internally.[29] Because of its unique size and chemical structure, lipoic acid works as an antioxidant that can penetrate both fat soluble (like vitamin E) and water soluble (like vitamin C) portions of the body.[30] This gives lipoic acid access to virtually the entire body, whereas most antioxidants only protect isolated areas of the body.

Lipoic acid also works to improve the efficiency of insulin by allowing blood glucose into the cells. Animal studies showed that supplements of lipoic acid increased insulin sensitivity by 30-50% and reduced plasma insulin and free fatty acids by 15-17%.[31]

Lipoic acid prevents "glycation" or glycosylation, which means the binding of sugar molecules to important proteins in the bloodstream, cell membrane, nerve tissue, etc. Glycation is a disastrous "tanning" that occurs, not unlike turning soft cow skin into hard leather in the tanning process. These new proteins that are bound to sugars do not have the same abilities as before the glycation process. Supplements of lipoic acid have been found to reverse the peripheral neuropathy from diabetes in as little as 3 weeks.[32] Lipoic acid improves blood flow to the nerves, which then improves nerve conduction.[33]

Lipoic acid increases the available levels of other antioxidants in the body, like vitamin E[34] and glutathione.[35] While there are many antioxidants found in a healthy diet and produced in the body (like uric acid), lipoic acid is the only antioxidant that meets the "wish list" of Dr. Lester Packer of the University of California at Berkeley. That "perfect" antioxidant should:

⇒ neutralize free radicals
⇒ be rapidly absorbed and quickly utilized by the body cells
⇒ be able to enhance the action of other antioxidants
⇒ be concentrated both inside and outside cells and cell membranes
⇒ promote normal gene expression
⇒ chelate metal ions, or drag toxic minerals out of the body.[36]

QUERCETIN

While a review paper from 1983 estimated that about 500 varieties of bioflavonoids existed in nature[37], more current estimates go as high as 20,000 different bioflavonoid compounds. Bioflavonoids are basically accessory factors used by plants to assist in photosynthesis and reduce the damaging effects from the sun. Best sources of bioflavonoids are citrus, berries, onions, parsley, legumes, green tea and bee pollen. The average Western diet contains somewhere between 150 mg/day[38] and 1000 mg/day[39] of bioflavonoids, with about 25 mg/day of quercetin. Best source of quercetin is the white rind in citrus fruits and onions. Quercetin has many talents that may help the diabetic patient:[40]

◊ Inhibits inflammation, by reducing histamine release
◊ Potent antioxidant
◊ Inhibits capillary fragility which protects connective tissue against breakdown
◊ Reduces the "stickiness" of cells, or aggregation, thus delaying stroke or heart disease

Quercetin has taught scientists a great lesson. Quercetin was considered a possible carcinogen based upon the Ames in vitro test in 1977, since it caused mutagenic changes to cells. Yet, new studies show that quercetin is not a carcinogen, but may be one of the most potent anticarcinogens in nature.[41]

One problem for diabetic patients can be inflammation, or swelling of tissue. Quercetin can help reduce swelling by helping to produce anti-inflammatory prostaglandins.[42] Quercetin inhibits the release of histamine from mast cells, thus reducing allergic reactions.[43] Quercetin also helps to stabilize cell membranes, decrease lipid peroxidation and inhibit the breakdown of connective tissue (collagen) by hyaluronidase (one of the ways that cancer spreads).[44]

GRAPE SEED EXTRACT 50 MG

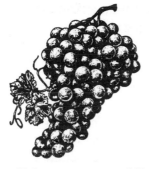

Scurvy (deficiency of vitamin C) has played a huge role in human history. Humans roamed the oceans of the world throughout the 15th through 19th century, often losing up to half of the people on board ship due to scurvy. The English physician, James Lind, discovered that limes cured scurvy in 1747 and began to wind down the death toll from scurvy, while also labelling the English sailors as "limeys". In 1930, Nobel prize winner, Albert Szent-Gyorgy, MD, PhD, isolated pure vitamin C. Ironically, the pure white crystalline vitamin C that Dr. Szent-Gyorgy isolated would not cure bleeding gums, whereas the crude brown mixture of citrus extract would. The difference between these two mixtures was "bioflavonoids", which include over 20,000 different chemical compounds that generally assist chlorophyll in photosynthesis and protect the plant from the harmful effects of the sun's radiation. The rainbow colors of fall foliage are Nature's art exhibit of bioflavonoids and carotenoids.

Some of the main categories of bioflavonoids include:
◊ anthocyanins; deep purple compounds found in black grapes, beets, red onions, and berries

◊ catechins and epigallocatechin, which are polyphenols found in apples and green
◊ ellagic acid, a true anti-cancer compound found in cranberries, raspberries, and other berries.
◊ flavones, found in citrus fruit, red grapes and green beans
◊ flavanols, such as quercetin, myricetin, found in kale, spinach, onions, apples, and black tea
◊ flavanones, such as hesperidin and naringen found in citrus fruits of grapefruit, oranges and lemons.

Some of the better known bioflavonoids include rutin, which is defined in the DORLAND'S MEDICAL DICTIONARY as capable of "preventing capillary fragility." Hesperidin, quercetin, pycnogenol from pine bark, and proanthocyanidins are other popular bioflavonoids. While bioflavonoids are known to be essential in the diet of insects, bioflavonoids are not yet considered essential in the human diet.

Proanthocyanidins can exist in a variety of forms, often referred to as grape seed extract. As the science of nutrition matures, we are finding that some of the "star" nutrients of the past may be just "supporting actors" for the real star nutrients. For instance, tocotrienols and Coenzyme Q may be more important than vitamin E in human health. Eicosapentaenoic acid (EPA from fish oil), though not considered essential, may be more important than alpha-linolenic acid (ALA from flax oil), which is considered essential. And bioflavonoids may be more important than vitamin C.

Bioflavonoids are potent chelators, helping to eliminate toxic minerals from the system.[45] Bioflavonoids in general help to reduce allergic reactions. OPC traps lipid peroxides, hydroxyl radicals, delays the onset of lipid peroxidation, prevents iron-induced lipid peroxidation, inhibits the enzymes that can degrade connective tissue (hyaluronidase, elastase, collagenase). Bioflavonoids may inhibit heart disease, stroke, and eye and nerve damage in diabetics.

L-CARNITINE 100-2000 MG

Think of carnitine as the "shoveller throwing fresh coals into the furnace" of the cell's mitochondria. Carnitine was first isolated from meat extracts in 1905, hence the "carnitine", refers to animal sources. Indeed, there is virtually no carnitine in plant foods, with red meats having the highest carnitine content.[46] The typical American diet provides from 5-100 mg/day of carnitine. Humans can manufacture carnitine in the liver and kidney from the precursors (raw materials to make) of lysine and methionine, and the cofactors of vitamin C, niacin, B-6 and iron. A deficiency of any of these precursors may lead to a carnitine deficiency, which involves buildup of fats in the blood, liver and muscles and may lead to symptoms of weakness--all of which is typical in poorly controlled diabetes. Since infants require carnitine in their diet and other individuals have been found to have clinical carnitine deficiencies, some nutritionists have lobbied to have carnitine included as an essential nutrient, not unlike niacin.[47]

Carnitine may help the diabetic patient by:
◊ protecting the liver from fatty buildup[48]
◊ improving energy and endurance[49]

Carnitine is probably essential in the diet for people who are very young, or sick, stressed, diabetic, older, burdened with toxins, etc.

HERBS

BITTER MELON

This cucumber-like plant grows throughout Asia, Africa, and South America and is widely hailed both in folk medicine circles and from scientific investigation for its ability to lower blood sugar levels. Two ounces of bitter melon juice improved blood glucose levels in 73% of Type 2 diabetics tested.[50] Another study gave 15 grams of extract from bitter melon to produce a 54% drop in after meal (post-prandial) blood glucose and 17% reduction in glycosylated hemoglobin.[51]

GYMNEMA SYLVESTRE

Gymnema sylvestre is a plant native to tropical regions of India and has a lengthy record of use in the treatment of both Type 1 and 2 diabetes. Giving Gymnema extract to Type 1 diabetics helped to reduce insulin requirements and improve blood glucose regulation.[52] When 400 mg/day of Gymnema extract was given to 22 patients with Type 2 diabetes along with their oral hypoglycemic drugs, all patients experienced improved blood glucose control and 5 of these subjects were able to discontinue drug usage altogether, using just Gymnema to regulate blood glucose.[53]

FENUGREEK

Once a spice and staple in southeastern Europe and western Asia, fenugreek seeds have long been used in folk medicine to treat diabetes. Today, we know scientifically that fenugreek seed powder is a potent agent for reducing levels of fats and glucose in the blood. Fairly hefty amounts of fenugreek, around 15-50 grams twice daily, are required to seriously lower blood sugar levels.[54] Since defatted fenugreek seed powder is a somewhat bitter substance, it usually requires the person to swallow it in capsules. 50 grams of capsules twice daily is a lot of work. Some people, especially east Indians, use fenugreek powder as a condiment, like we use salt, which makes its use as a supplement much more realistic.

SALT BUSH

Salt bush is a plant native to the Middle East. Researchers in Israel found that 3 grams daily of salt bush capsules provided improved blood glucose regulation in Type 2 diabetes.

BILBERRY

European blueberry, or bilberry, has been used in France since 1945 to treat diabetic retinopathy. A mixture of bioflavonoids in bilberry both reduce blood glucose levels and also protect the macula of the diabetic's eye. Several studies have found enhanced vision in diabetics using bilberry supplements of 80-160 mg three times daily.

GINKGO BILOBA (24% HETEROSIDE) 40 MG

The ginkgo tree is one of the oldest living species on earth, having been around for over 200 million years. The ginkgo tree is an incredibly adaptable and tenacious plant. One ginkgo tree survived the near-ground zero nuclear blast in Hiroshima, Japan. There are now over 1,000 scientific studies published over the past 40 years demonstrating the medicinal value of ginkgo, with ginkgo extract becoming one of the more widely prescribed medications in Europe today. In 1989, over 100,000 physicians worldwide wrote over 10 million prescriptions for ginkgo.

There are several ways in which ginkgo may help the diabetic patient:

◊ Vasodilator, expands the tiny capillaries that nourish 90% of the body's tissues, thus bringing oxygen and nutrients to the cells. In doing so, ginkgo improves depression[55] and general circulation to the organs, while reducing the risk for heart disease.[56]

◊ Inhibits platelet aggregation, or the stickiness of cells. Stroke and heart attacks are fueled by sticky cells which are generated by Platelet Activating Factor (PAF). Ginkgo inhibits PAF.[57] By modifying PAF, ginkgo helps to reduce inflammation and allergic responses.[58]

◊ Antioxidant of exceptional efficiency.[59] Slows down free radical destruction of healthy tissue, therefore protects blood vessel walls, lens and macula of the eyes, nerves and other tissue that normally is exposed to a storm of free radical destruction in the diabetic.

GLUCOSOL
EXTRACT FROM LAGERSTROEMIA SPECIOSA L.

In a placebo controlled cross over study with 24 diabetic subjects in Japan, corosolic acid (the active ingredient) in the proprietary product Glucosol (available at health food stores) was able to lower blood glucose levels by about 14%, a modest but well documented result.

GINSENG

Ginseng is one of the world's oldest herbs, used by many cultures over the past 5,000 years. Ginseng is one of the classical "adaptogens", which is an elite group of herbs that improve various aspects of the bodily processes. If a person has high blood pressure, then ginseng will often help to lower it toward normal. If a person has low blood pressure, then ginseng will often help to raise it to normal. No drug has such an unexplainable ability to alter the body's processes in whatever direction they need to go.

In a double blind study, 36 Type 2 diabetics were given either placebo, 100 mg ginseng, or 200 mg ginseng. The diabetics who received ginseng had measurable improvements in mood, body weight, and blood sugar levels. The group that received the highest dosage of ginseng, 200 mg, also had improvements in glycosylated hemoglobin, a sign that blood glucose levels have slowed the destructive "tanning" of blood proteins.

PATIENT PROFILE

J.W. got very lucky. She developed Type 2 diabetes in her 60s and needed hypoglycemic drugs to control her blood glucose levels. And yet she was diagnosed healthy and non-diabetic within 4 months after starting my program. She asked me:"Which of these foods and nutrients will give me the biggest 'bang for my buck' in reversing my diabetes." I recommended supplements of lipoic acid, bitter melon, chromium, Gymnema sylvestre, vitamins E & C; while adding to her diet flax oil, brewer's yeast, vinegar, onions, fish, and lots of cinnamon. Her compliance was amazing and she was very appreciative of her returned better health.

ENDNOTES

[1] . Vahouny, G, et al., DIETARY FIBER IN HEALTH AND DISEASE, Plenum, NY, 1982

[2] . Simpson, HR, et al., Lancet, vol.1, p.1, 1981

[3] . Jenkins, DJA, et al., Am.J.Clin.Nutr., vol.33, p.1729, 1980

[4] . Cunningham, J, Metabolism, vol.40, p.146, 1991

[5] . Davie, SJ, et al., Diabetes, vol.41, p.167, 1992

[6] . Cleary, JP, J.Nutr.Med., vol.1, p.217, 1990

[7] . Maebashi, M., et al., J.Clin.Biochem.Nutr., vol.14, p.211, 1993

[8] . Jones, CL, et al., J.Am.Pod.Assoc., vol.68, p.646, 1978

[9] . Coelingh-Bennick, HJT, et al., Br.Med.J., vol.3, p.13, 1975

[10] . Sancetta, SM, et al., Ann.Int.Med., vol.35, p.1028, 1951

[11] . Bhatt, HR, et al., Lancet, vol.2, p.572, 1983

[12] . Paolisso, G., et al., Am.J.Clin.Nutr., vol.61, p.848, 1995

[13] . Salonen, JT, Br.Med.J., vol.311, p. 1124, 1995

[14] . Anderson, R. et al., Diabetes, vol.45, p.124A, suppl2, 1996

[15] . White, JR, et al., Ann.Pharmacother., vol.27, p.775, 1993

[16]. Forbes, GB, in PRESENT KNOWLEDGE IN NUTRITION, p.11, International Life Sciences Institute, Washington, 1996

[17] . Mindell, EL, THE MSM MIRACLE, p.10, Keats, New Canaan, 1997

[18] . Jacob, SW, et al., Ann.NY.Acad.Sci., vol.441, p.13, 1983

[19] . Morton, JI, et al., Proc.Soc.Exp.Med., vol.183, no.2, p.227, Nov.1986

[20] . Keen, CL, et al., in PRESENT KNOWLEDGE IN NUTRITION, p.339, ILSI, Washington, 1996

[21] . Harland, BF, et al., J.Am.Diet.Assoc., vol.94, p.891, 1994

[22] . Cohen, N., et al., J.Clin.Invest., vol.95, p.2501, 1995

[23] . Brichard, SM, et al., Trends Pharmacol.Sci., vol.16, p.265, 1995

[24] . Riel, RR, J.Dairy Sci., vol.46, p.102, 1963

[25] . Sebedio, JL, et al., Biochimica et Biophysica Acta, vol.1345, p.5, 1997

[26] . Houseknecht, KL, et al., Biochem. Biophys.Res.Commun., vol.244, p.678, 1998

[27] . Decker, EA, Nutrition Reviews, vol.53, no.3, p.49, Mar.1995

[28]. Budavari, S. (eds), THE MERCK INDEX, p.1591, Merck & Co., Whitehouse Station, NJ 1996

[29]. Packer, L., et al., Free Radical Biol. Med., vol.19, p.227, 1995

[30]. Stoll, S., et al., Ann.NY Acad.Sci., vol.717, p.122, 1994

[31]. Jacob, S., et al., Diabetes, vol.45, p.1024, 1996

[32]. Passwater, R., LIPOIC ACID, Keats, New Canaan, CT, 1996

[33]. Nagamatsu, M., et al., Diabetes Care, vol.18, p.1160, Aug.1995

[34]. Podda, M., et al., Biochem.Biophys., Res.Commun., vol.204, p.98, 1994

[35]. Han, D., et al., Biochem.Biophys.,Res.Commun., vol.207, p.258, 1995

[36]. Ou, P., et al., Biochem.Pharmacol., vol.50, p.123, 1995

[37]. Havsteen, B., Biochem.Pharmacol., vo.32, p.1141, 1983

[38]. Murray, MT, ENCYCLOPEDIA OF NUTRITIONAL SUPPLEMENTS, p.321, Prima, Rocklin, CA 1996

[39]. Middleton, E., et al., in ADJUVANT NUTRITION IN CANCER TREATMENT, Quillin, P. (eds), p.319, Cancer Treatment Research Foundation, Arlington Heights, IL 1994

[40]. Boik, J., CANCER & NATURAL MEDICINE, p.181, Oregon Medical Press, Princeton, MN 1995

[41]. Stavric, B., Clin.Biochem., vol.27, p.245, Aug.1994

[42]. Bauman, J., et al., Prostaglandins, vol.20, p.627, 1980

[43]. Middleton, E, et al., Arch.Allergy Appl.Immunol., vol.77, p.155, 1985

[44]. Busse, WW, et al., J.Allergy Clin.Immunol., vol.73, p.801, 1984

[45]. Havsteen, B, Biochem Pharmacol., vol.32, p.1141, 1983

[46]. Bremer, J., Physiol.Rev., vol.63, p.1420, 1983

[47]. Borum, PR, et al., J.Am.Coll.Nutr., vol.5, p.177, 1986

[48]. Sachan, DS, et al., Am.J.Clin.Nutr., vol.39, p.738, 1984

[49]. Dragan, GI, et al., Physiologie, vol.25, p.231, 1987

[50]. Welihinda, J., et al., J.Ethnopharmacol., vol.17, p.277, 1986

[51]. Srivastava, Y, et al., Phytotherapy Res., vol.7, p.285, 1993

[52]. Shanmugasundaram, ERB, et al., J.Ethnopharmacol., vol.30, p.281, 1990

[53]. Baskaran, K., et al., J.Ethnopharmacol., vol.30, p.295, 1990

[54]. Mada, Z., et al., Eur.J.Clin.Nutr., vol.42, p.51, 1988

[55]. Schubert, H., et al., Geriatr Forsch, vol.3, p.45, 1993

[56]. Kleijnen, J., et al., Br. J. Clin.Pharmacol. vol.34, p.352, 1992

[57]. Kleijnen, J., et al., Lancet, vol.340, p.1136, 1992

[58]. Koltai, M., et al., Drugs, vol.42, p.9, 1991

[59]. Pincemail, J., et al., Experientia, vol.45, p.708, 1989

CHAPTER 9

CHANGING THE UNDERLYING CAUSES OF DIABETES

ADDITIONAL THERAPIES THAT MAY HELP DIABETICS

"No one with a headache is suffering from a deficiency of aspirin." anonymous

> Help reverse diabetes by changing the underlying causes of the disease. These are listed in approximate order of importance. Find a health care professional who will help you detect and solve these problems.

Few Type 2 diabetics have a deficiency of insulin or hypoglycemic drugs in their system. No one with elevated serum cholesterol is suffering from a deficiency of clofibrate. Arthritis sufferers are not suffering due to lack of cortisone, and cancer patients are not lacking chemotherapy. All of these therapies are short term, symptom-fixing drugs which provide immediate relief, but do nothing to change the underlying causes of a disease.

Studies have proven that patients who undergo coronary bypass surgery have no extension in lifespan, because no one has changed the cause of the disease by replacing 4 inches of

COMMON PATHOGENIC CONDITIONS

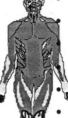

- Psycho-spiritual
- Toxic burden
- Malnutrition
- Exercise
- Blood glucose
- Redox
- Immune dysfunction
- Gland/organ insufficiency

- Maldigestion
- Chronic infections
- pH
- Hypoxia
- Effects of aging
- Physical alignment
- Energy alignment
- Mechanical injury

plugged up "plumbing" or arteries near the heart. Same goes for other drugs and conditions. Beta-blockers and diuretics for the 60 million Americans with high blood pressure actually INCREASE the risk for a heart attack by causing a loss of the crucial cardio-protective minerals of potassium and magnesium.

The following listing is a very brief description of the underlying causes of disease, listed in order of importance (my professional opinion). These biological, psychological, chemical and electrical factors have been gleaned and synthesized from such classic works as THE TEXTBOOK OF NATURAL MEDICINE by Drs. Pizzorno and Murray, and OPTIMAL WELLNESS by Dr. Ralph Golan. The ideal combination therapy for any disease would include short term relief with minimal drugs, coupled with the long term goal of changing the underlying causes of the disease. For more information, consult with your health care professional. Naturopathic Doctors (ND) are usually well trained in these theories.

FIX WHAT'S BROKE

If you have a zinc deficiency, then a truckload of vitamin C will not be nearly as valuable as giving the body what it needs to end the zinc deficiency. If an accumulation of lead and mercury has crimped the immune system, then removing the toxic metals is more important than psychotherapy. If a low output of hydrochloric acid in the stomach creates poor digestion and malabsorption, then hydrochloric acid supplements are the answer. If a broken spirit brought on the diabetes, then spiritual healing is necessary to eliminate the diabetes.

The need to "fix what's broke" is a prime limiting factor in studies that examine diabetic therapies. In a given group of 100 diabetic patients, based upon my experience, 80 may need counseling to help them with their eating disorder which has generated obesity, 60 may need high dose supplements of fish oil, chromium and others to rectify problems in the insulin receptor on the cell membrane, 5 may need serious detoxification, and 75 have a complex combination of problems. This issue complicates diabetic treatment tremendously and makes "cookbook" diabetic treatment an exercise in futility. Our progress against diabetes has been crippled not only by the complexity of the disease, but also by the need for Western science to isolate one variable. We will eventually help most diabetic patients by fixing whatever bodily function needs repair. This is easier said than done. Finding the underlying problem requires a physician trained in comprehensive medicine.

1) PSYCHO-SPIRITUAL.

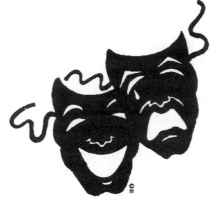

Grief, loss of loved one, lack of purpose, depression, low self esteem, hypochondriasis as means of attention, needing love for ourself and others, touching, be here now, sense of accomplishment, happiness, music, beauty, sexual satisfaction, forgiveness, etc..

Researchers at the National Institute of Health, spearheaded by Candice Pert, PhD, have investigated the link between catecholamines, endorphins and other chemicals from the brain.

The good news is that the mind can be a powerful instrument at controlling stress, overeating, and beginning an exercise program. This "personal responsibility" is a frightening or empowering concept, depending on how you chose to perceive it. Helplessness and hopelessness are just as lethal as cigarettes and bullets.

Enkephalins and endorphins, also called "the mind's rivers of pleasure", are brain chemicals that are secreted when the mind is happy. Endorphins improve the general functioning of the body and blood glucose levels. Depending on your attitude, your mind either encourages or discourages disease in your body.

The take-home lesson here is: you can take a soup bowl full of potent nutrients to fight diabetes while you are being treated by the world's best endocrinologist; but if your mind is not happy and focused on the need for peace and forgiveness in life, then the previous program of nutrition will not be nearly as effective as it should be.

2) TOXIC BURDEN.

INTAKE from voluntary pollutants of drugs, alcohol, tobacco. Involuntary toxins from food, water, & air.
>SOLUTION: DETOXIFICATION (EXCRETION) VIA urine, feces, sweat, liver, other. Some chose chelation therapy, mercury amalgam removal, magnets to neutralize EMF pollution.

3) MALNUTRITION

All creatures on earth are heavily dependent on our nutrient intake for health, vitality, disease resistance, and longevity. See the chapter on malnutrition in America for details.

4) EXERCISE.

Exercise plays a huge role in preventing, controlling, and reversing diabetes. Humans evolved as active creatures. Our biochemical processes depend on regular exercise to maintain homeostasis. A well respected Stanford physician, Dr. William Bortz, published a review of the scientific literature on exercise and concluded: "our dis-eases may be from dis-use of the body."[1] Exercise stabilizes blood sugar levels and brings oxygen to the body. The most essential nutrient in the human body is oxygen. Westerners typically are sedentary and breath shallowly, which deprives the body of oxygen.

Exercise is an absolutely essential ingredient for the diabetic's health. A primary tool for detoxification, stabilizing blood glucose levels, improving digestion and regularity, proper oxygenation of tissue, stress tolerance, improving hormone output (i.e. growth hormone & DHEA), burning fatty tissue, eliminating harmful by-products (i.e., estrogen, uric acid). A wide variety of studies have shown that most diabetics benefit tremendously when incorporating a decent exercise program of 30 minutes each day.

5) BLOOD GLUCOSE

Elevations in blood glucose play havoc on the human body. See the chapter on "glucotoxicity"; killing us sweetly.

6) REDOX

Life is a continuous balancing act between oxidative forces (pro-oxidants) and protective forces (antioxidants). We want to fully oxygenate the tissue, which generates pro-oxidants, but we also want to protect healthy tissue from excess oxidative destruction, using antioxidants. Antioxidants are a sacrificial substance, to be destroyed in lieu of body tissue. Antioxidants include beta-carotene, C, E, selenium, zinc, riboflavin, manganese, cysteine, methionine, N-acetylcysteine, and many herbal extracts (i.e. green tea, pycnogenols, curcumin). Diabetics need more antioxidants than non-diabetic people.

7) IMMUNE DYSFUNCTIONS

We have an extensive network of protective factors that circulate throughout our bodies to kill any bacteria, virus, yeast or cancer cells. Think of these 20 trillion immune cells as both your Department of Defense and your waste disposal company. The immune system of the average American is "running on empty" and the diabetic is even more trouble. Causes for this problem include toxic burden, stress, no exercise, poor diet, unbridled use of antibiotics and vaccinations, innoculations from world travelers, and less breast feeding.

8) GLAND OR ORGAN INSUFFICIENCY

As we age, many glands and organs produce less vital hormones and secretions: including the stomach (hydrochloric acid), pancreas (digestive enzymes), thyroid (thyroxin), adrenals (DHEA, cortisol), thymus (thymic extract), spleen

(spleen concentrate), joints (glucosamine sulfate), pineal (melatonin), and pituitary (growth hormone).

Replacing missing secretions often dramatically improves health. Since 90% of Type 2 diabetics are obese and hypothyroidism often manifests itself as obesity, the diabetic needs screening for hypothyroidism to rule this out as an underlying cause of the disease.

9) MALDIGESTION

After a lifetime of high fat, high sugar, overeating, too much alcohol, stress, drugs, indigestible foods (i.e., pizza); many Americans have poor peristalsis, insufficient stomach and intestinal secretions, damaged microvilli, imbalances of friendly (probiotic) vs unfriendly (anaerobic, pathogenic) bacteria. One must remove, repair, replace, re-inoculate. Food separation (combinations) may be of value for a brief time until the GI tract recuperates. Digestive enzymes and/or hydrochloric acid taken with meals may help.

10) CHRONIC INFECTIONS.

Many American suffer from chronic systemic yeast and bacterial infections, and even intestinal parasites.

11) pH (potential hydrogens)

Acid alkaline balance (7.41 ideal in human veins) brought about by proper breathing, exercise (carbonic buffer from carbon dioxide in blood), diet (plant foods elevate pH, animal foods and sugar reduce pH), water (adequate hydration improves pH), other agents, such as cesium chloride, citric acid, sodium bicarbonate

12) HYPOXIA

Humans are aerobic organisms. All cells thrive when there is proper oxygenation to the tissue. Red blood cell production is dependent on iron, copper, B-6, folate, B-12, protein, & zinc. Adequate exercise and proper breathing help. Cofactors, like CoQ, B-vitamins improve aerobic energy metabolism in cell mitochondria. Fatty acids in diet dictate "membrane fluidity" of all cells and ability to absorb oxygen.

13) EFFECTS OF AGING.

By age 65, the average American has eaten 100,000 lb (50 tons) of food. Poor diet accumulates in chronic sub-clinical malnutrition; such as calcium & osteoporosis, chromium & diabetes, vitamin E & heart disease, vitamin C and cancer. Toxins accumulate in fatty tissue and liver. Chronic exposure to unchecked pro-oxidants eventually creates diabetes, arthritis, Alzheimer's, heart disease, stroke, cancer, etc. Organ reserve is used up in stress and poor diet. The Hayflick principle tells us that we have 55 cell divisions maximum in a lifetime. Once your "bank account" is empty, it is difficult to recover from serious disease. Errors in DNA replication become more common as we age. Telomeres become shortened. The risk for diabetes doubles after age 40.

14) PHYSICAL ALIGNMENT

Spinal vertebrae must be in proper alignment. Chiropractic & osteopathic manipulations on spine, joints, skull plates can be helpful. Accidents, poor muscle tone, and aging create alignment problems. Nerves and blood vessels radiate from the spinal column which can become misaligned and cause compression on these vital channels of energy. Exercise, inversion and physical manipulations from chiropractic or osteopathic physicians may solve these problems.

15) ENERGY ALIGNMENT

Meridians, shakras, and energy pathways were discovered by acupuncturists. Use magnets, acupuncture, electro-acupuncture, and acupressure to correct these problems. Homeopathy probably works on this level.

16) MECHANICAL INJURY

Chronic injury requires hyperplasia, or the growth of new cells. If not properly nourished, new cell growth can become erratic and error-prone.

PATIENT PROFILE

B. J. was forced by his wife to go to the doctor. His "heartburn" had become so frequent and interrupted too many otherwise pleasant meals with the family. B.J.'s doctor put him on the drug, Tagamet, and his condition seemed to disappear. However, at his next physical, B.J. showed up with high blood pressure at the tender age of 46. His doctor put him on beta-blockers and diuretics and the blood pressure came down. A year later, B.J. started developing severe depression from the impotence that resulted from his high blood pressure medication. His doctor started him on Prozac for that symptom. B.J.'s doctor also prescribed medication for his swollen and tender joints, corticosteroids, that sent his blood sugar levels into full blown Type 2 diabetes. This "shell game" of "hide the symptoms with drugs" continued for a few more years until B.J. started passing blood in his stools and was diagnosed with colon cancer. No one had bothered to ask the simple but essential question: "What is causing these conditions?" In B.J.'s case, a very poor on-the-run diet that was deficient in many nutrients, plus stress, no exercise and the side effects of excess medication came crashing down in a really serious life threatening condition. Find the underlying cause of your diabetes for a long term favorable outcome in your disease.

ENDNOTES

[1]. Bortz, WM, Journal American Medical Association, vol.248, no.10, p.1203, Sept.10, 1982

APPENDIX

GOOD NUTRITION REFERENCES:

Anderson, WELLNESS MEDICINE, Keats, 1987

Balch & Balch, PRESCRIPTION FOR NUTRITIONAL HEALING, Avery, 1993

Eaton, PALEOLITHIC PRESCRIPTION, Harper & Row, 1988

Grabowski, RJ, CURRENT NUTRITIONAL THERAPY, Image Press, 1993

Haas, STAYING HEALTHY WITH NUTRITION, Celestial, 1992

Hausman, THE RIGHT DOSE, Rodale, 1987

Hendler, DOCTOR'S VITAMIN AND MINERAL ENCYCLOPEDIA, Simon & Schuster,1990

Lieberman, S. et al., REAL VITAMIN & MINERAL BOOK, Avery, 1990

Murray, M, et al., ENCYCLOPEDIA OF NATURAL MEDICINE, Prima, 1990

National Research Council, RECOMMENDED DIETARY ALLOWANCES, Nat Academy, 1989

Price, NUTRITION AND PHYSICAL DEGENERATION, Keats, 1989

Quillin, P., HEALING NUTRIENTS, Random House, 1987

Shils, ME, et al., MODERN NUTRITION IN HEALTH & DISEASE, Lea & Febiger, 1994

Werbach, M, NUTRITIONAL INFLUENCES ON ILLNESS, Third Line, 1993

WHERE TO BUY NUTRITION PRODUCTS BY MAIL ORDER

BULK FOODS

Allergy Resources Inc., 195 Huntington Beach Dr., Colorado Springs, CO 80921, ph 719-488-3630

Deer Valley Farm, RD#1, Guilford, NY 13780, ph. 607-674-8556

Diamond K Enterprises, Jack Kranz, R.R. 1, Box 30, St. Charles, MN 55972, ph. 507-932-4308

Gravelly Ridge Farms, Star Route 16, Elk Creek, CA 95939, ph. 916-963-3216

Green Earth, 2545 Prairie St., Evanston, IL 60201, ph. 800-322-3662

Healthfoods Express, 181 Sylmar Clovis, CA 93612, ph. 209-252-8321

Jaffe Bros. Inc., PO Box 636, Valley Center, CA 92082, ph. 619-749-1133

Macrobiotic Wholesale Co., 799 Old Leicester Hwy, Asheville, NC 28806, ph. 704-252-1221

Moksha Natural Foods, 724 Palm Ave., Watsonville, CA, 95076, ph. 408-724-2009

Mountain Ark Co., 120 South East Ave., Fayetteville, AR, 72701, ph. 501-442-7191, or 800-643-8909

New American Food Co., PO Box 3206, Durham, NC 27705, ph. 919-682-9210

Timber Crest Farms, 4791 Dry Creek, Healdsburg, CA, 95448, ph. 707-433-8251, FAX -8255

Walnut Acres, Walnut Acres Road, Penns Creek, PA 17862, ph. 717-837-0601

LARGE STORES THAT SELL VITAMINS, MINERALS, & SOME HERBS BY MAIL

NutriGuard, 800-433-2402

Health Center for Better Living, 813-566-2611

Vitamin Research Products, 800-877-2447

Vitamin Trader, 800-334-9310

Willner Chemists, 800-633-1106

STORES THAT SPECIALIZE IN SELLING HERBS BY MAIL
Gaia Herbals, 800-994-9355
Frontier Herbs 800-786-1388; fax 319-227-7966
Blessed Herbs 800-489-HERB; fax 508-882-3755
Trout Lake Farm 509-395-2025
San Francisco Herb Co. fax 800-227-5430
Star West 800-800-4372

RECOMMENDED COOKBOOKS
Super Seafood, Tom Ney
Eat Well, Live Well, Pamela Smith
Natural Foods Cookbook, Mary Estella
The Healthy Gourmet Cookbook, Barbara Bassett
How to Use Natural Foods Deliciously, Barbara Bassett
Eat Smart for a Healthy Heart Cookbook, Dr. Denton Cooley
Simply Light Cooking, Kitchens of Weight Watchers
Healthy Life-Style Cookbook, Weight Watchers
The American Health Food Book, Robert Barnett, Nao Hauser
The Chez Eddy Living Heart Cookbook, Antonio Gotto Jr.

DIABETES SUPPORT ORGANIZATIONS
American Diabetes Association, 1660 Duke St., Alexandria, VA
22314; ph.800-342-2383; www.diabetes.org
Canadian Diabetes Association, 15 Toronto St. #1001, Toronto,
Ontario M5C 2E3, ph.416-363-3373, www.diabetes.ca
Central Diabetes Program, US Indian Health Services, 5300
Homestead Rd NE, Albuquerque, NM 87110, ph.505-248-4182;
www.tucson.his.gov
Centers for Disease Control, TISB Mail Stop K-13, 4770 Buford
Hwy NE, Atlanta, GA 30341-3724, ph.770-488-5080
Juvenile Diabetes Foundation, 120 Wall St., NY, NY 10005, ph.800-
533-2873; www.jdfcure.com
Taking Control of your Diabetes, 149 Seventh St., Del Mar, CA
92014; ph 619-755-5683; www.tcoyd.com

Honey, Garlic and Vinegar Better Than Prescription Drugs?

(SPECIAL) We know from scholars that ancient civilizations relied on their healing power for a wide variety of ailments. In fact, honey was so prized by the Romans for its medicinal properties that it was sometimes used instead of gold to pay taxes. Egyptian doctors believed garlic was the ultimate cure-all. And vinegar is said to have been used for everything from arthritis to obesity for thousands of years.

Today doctors and researchers hail the healing abilities of honey, garlic and vinegar as much more than folklore. Hundreds of scientific studies have been conducted on this dream team of healers. The results are conclusive on their amazing power to help many common health problems.

These studies prove that this trio from nature's pharmacy can help **reduce blood pressure, lower cholesterol, improve circulation and lower blood sugar levels.** Scientific evidence also indicates that they may be of some value in the treatment of: **arthritis, athlete's foot, bronchitis, burns, colds and flu, cold sores, constipation, cramps, diarrhea, eczema, earaches, fatigue, fungus, heart problems, muscle aches, rheumatism, ringworm, sinus congestion, sore throat, urinary infections, virus and yeast infections and more.**

An amazing book called *Honey, Garlic & Vinegar Home Remedies* is now available to the general public. It shows you exactly how to make hundreds of remedies using honey, garlic and vinegar separately and in unique combinations. Each preparation is carefully described along with the health condition for which it is formulated .

Learn how to prepare ointments, tonics, lotions, poultices, syrups and compresses in your own kitchen. Whip up a batch to treat:
- **CORNS & CALLOUSES:** Get rid of them fast with this natural method
- **HEADACHE:** Enjoy fast relief without drugs
- **HEMORRHOIDS:** Don't suffer another day without this proven recipe
- **LEG CRAMPS:** Try this simple way to quick relief
- **MUSCLE ACHES:** Just mix up a batch of this and rub it on
- **STINGS & BITES:** Medical journals recommend this remedy to reduce pain and swelling fast
- **STOMACH PROBLEMS:** This remedy calms upset stomach and is noted in a medical journal for ulcers
- **TOOTHACHE:** This remedy can give relief until you can get to the dentist
- **WEIGHT LOSS:** Secret remedy speeds fat burn and flushes stubborn fat from hiding places

Discover all these health tips and more. You'll find: ***Dozens of easy-to-make beauty preparations for hair and skin, including a wrinkle smoother that really works. *Loads of delicious recipes using these health-giving super foods. *Tons of money-saving cleaning compounds to keep your home, car and clothing sparkling.**

Right now, as part of a special introductory offer, you can receive a special press run of the book *Honey, Garlic & Vinegar Home Remedies* for only $8.95 plus $1.00 postage and handling. Your satisfaction is <u>100% guaranteed</u>. You must be completely satisfied, or simply return it in 90 days for a <u>full refund — no questions asked</u>.

HERE'S HOW TO ORDER: Simply print your name and address and the word "Remedies" on a piece of paper and mail it along with a check or money order for only $9.95 to: THE LEADER CO., INC., Publishing Division, Dept. HG101, P.O. Box 8347, Canton, Ohio 44711. (Make checks payable to The Leader Co., Inc.) VISA or MasterCard send card number and expiration date. Act now. Orders are filled on a first-come, first-served basis.

Plain Old Baking Soda A Drugstore In A Box?

Medical science recognizes the medicinal value of baking soda. For example, it is used in kidney dialysis to reduce levels of acids in the bloodstream. But there are hundreds of everyday uses for baking soda you've never heard of. They're all in a new book, now available to the general public, by contributing editor to Family Circle Magazine, Vicki Lansky.

Discover over 500 remedies using baking soda with other ordinary household items like: vinegar, lemon, toothpaste, sugar, salt and more. A little baking soda with a pinch of this and a dash of that can:

- **Soothe SORE GUMS, CANKER SORES and SUNBURN**
- **Make a SORE THROAT feel better**
- **Fight HEARTBURN and ACID INDIGESTION**
- **Ease the pain of BEE STINGS and BLISTERS**
- **Help PSORIASIS sufferers**
- **Dry up ACNE and POISON IVY**
- **Clear up a STUFFY NOSE and ITCHY EYES**
- **Replace lost salts from DIARRHEA**
- **Help relieve VAGINAL ITCHING**
- **Treat ATHLETE'S FOOT naturally**
- **STOP SMOKING naturally**

Can you believe that a baking soda formula was used to clean the interior of the Statue of Liberty in her recent restoration? Well, there's practically nothing under the sun that a baking soda recipe can't clean – and clean and deodorize better than expensive store-bought products. Fact is, baking soda is the ultimate deodorizer because it doesn't simply cover up odors – it actually absorbs them. It's a natural alternative to toxic, harsh chemical cleaners. Just whip up an easy baking soda recipe to make:

- **A powerful bleaching formula for formica**
- **Homemade scouring powder**
- **Drain cleaner for clogged drains**
- **Dishwasher detergent that makes dishes gleam**
- **An oven cleaner that eliminates elbow grease**
- **Allergy-free deodorizers for the whole house**
- **Upholstery cleaner that makes fabrics look new**
- **A cleaner for copper pot bottoms**
- **A great rust remover formula**
- **Tile cleanser that works like magic**
- **A little-known formula that really cleans old, porous tubs**
- **A lifesaver for white rings and spots on wood furniture**
- **The perfect cleaner for gold, silver and pearl jewelry**
- **A tooth whitener that makes teeth sparkle**
- **A denture soak that works great**

Imagine, over 500 time and money-saving tips like how to use baking soda to: melt ice on sidewalks, boost bleach's whitening power, remove age stains from linens, remove crayon and ink stains, keep icing moist, keep color in vegetables, make cuts disappear from countertops, clean stainless sinks without scratching, whiten porcelain sinks, put out grease and electrical fires, clean burned pans, clean up pet stains, eliminate gas from baked beans and the list goes on and on. There are even dozens of tips for around the garage like: how to remove bugs and tar from car, make a great car wash solution, unclog radiators, neutralize battery corrosion.

NOTES

NOTES

NOTES

NOTES